MW00774006

Able-Bodied Like Me

NAVIGATING & BALANCING CULTURES FROM THE SEAT OF MY PANTS

Matt Glowacki

© 2018 Matt Glowacki
All rights reserved.

ISBN: 0692052887
ISBN 13: 9780692052884
Library of Congress Control Number: 2018900298
Matt Glowacki, Sun Prairie, WI

Table of Contents

Author's Note

The truth and personal history I share in this book are my own as a disabled person. It is my personal narrative; I am aware of the privilege and position I am claiming in telling my story. It is my hope that my stories can serve as a bridge to bring people together in spirit and understanding. But they are not typical examples for people with disabilities.

In most cases, the details of the stories I share are reported from notes taken by me directly after the experiences and confirmed by parties involved. All other representations are my best recollections from my own memories and perspectives I have gained through my experiences.

Many of the people referenced in this book have given me their permission to share their names, stories, and truths. Where appropriate, I have changed a few small details to protect their personal privacy. When I share information and behavior about unnamed people and strangers, it is my intention to leave them anonymous to protect them from other people's judgments and to use their stories for educational purposes only.

I understand that labels are often used ignorantly and conscious word choice is appropriate in telling stories and in conveying ideas. I use "person with a disability" or "person with disabilities" as the primary means of description for my inclusive membership in my minority group. All other usage of linking inclusive language are meant not to offend, just to vary word choices and possibly reinforce the points being made in an illustration or to reinforce a persuasive argument.

"Real isn't how you were made;
it is the thing that happens to you."
The Velveteen Rabbit- Margery Williams

"Give Him a Chance to Surprise You"

The day of my birth affected my parents in a way that would forever change how they looked at the world. My mother's pregnancy with me was very typical. She had the cravings that mothers have: pickles and ice cream; the 2:00 AM craving for potato chips. Because she was pregnant during the early 1970s, she didn't have access to the sonogram technology common in today's world. Until my birth, nobody knew my legs didn't develop in the womb and the experts still have no good answer as to why I don't have them. They just claim it to be "one of those things."

When my older sister was born, the fathers of the newborns were not allowed to be in the delivery room with their spouse. But because of a policy change in the years since then, my father was allowed to play a supportive role in the hospital room when my mom gave birth to me. Everything was progressing as expected and there were smiles all around...until that changed. Suddenly the doctor and nurses' faces had expressions of concern. Mom asked, "Is there something wrong?"

The answer was "Yes."

Second question: "Can it be fixed?"

The answer was "No."

With concern, my mother asked, "Will the child live?"

The answer was "We're not sure."

"What's wrong?" my dad asked, seeing the doctor's face.

The doctor looked my father in the eye. "Your son is missing his legs."

Later, after the nurses cleaned me up and my parents met me, the doctor returned to check up on the new addition to the Glowacki family.

"I guess we'll have to sell the house," my dad said to the doctor.

The doctor was confused. "Why would you sell your home?"

My father explained to him that they had just completed construction on their dream home, a tri-level. There were seven stairs between each floor, and now he had a child without legs.

Many years later, as my dad recounted this story to me, he shared that immediately his mind was flooded with thoughts of the other problems that I would be facing in the new home—and he began to tell them to the doctor. But the doctor stopped him, interrupting with perhaps the best advice he could offer.

"Don't sell the house. Give him a chance to surprise you!"

That one sentence would forever change my family's expectations of me. What the doctor said laid the groundwork for a different outlook at the challenges I would face for the rest of my life.

Every perceived barrier was transformed into an opportunity. It became our family's mission to determine what I could do as opposed to what I couldn't. It wasn't always perfect—we went down a couple of incorrect roads because of the good intentions of others. Nevertheless, in the end, what mattered most was working with the challenges of not having legs and learning from the experience.

As you listen to my story and internalize my writing, my hope is that you will do your best to leave behind any preconceived notions of people with disabilities. I am asking you to do the same thing that my first doctor asked of my parents—to simply give me a chance to surprise you.

PART 1
Look Ma, No Legs!

CHAPTER 1

"I Would Have to Kill Myself..."

n 1973, I was born without legs, but it wasn't until 2014 that I realized I had a disability. I had to use prosthetics, and then a wheelchair, but I pay those no mind. My mode of transportation is just who I am. I refuse to see myself as disabled, or as any less than everyone else.

However, many times a week, as I am working, shopping, or just out and about, people stop and compliment me on how well I am doing in my "situation" and how I am a motivation to them. I always explain to them how happy that makes me to be able to inspire them, but I ask them to please understand that I am just doing what I need to do and getting done what I need to get done that day, just like them.

I know they believe they are paying me a compliment, but from my point of view, the conversation often goes downhill from there. It usually devolves into the stranger saying, "You are an inspiration to me. This morning when I got up, I was feeling really bad about myself...but then I saw you."

I sometimes look at them and respond, "You know, that isn't really a compliment."

They often look a little confused, but then they deliver the knockout blow: "No really, if I was like you, not having any legs and having to use a wheelchair, I would have to kill myself."

The first hundred times strangers said this to me, I was aghast. For someone to think the quality of my life was so poor, that my best day was so horrible it couldn't come close to justifying them wanting to be alive in my condition, was a bit disheartening.

It forced me to develop a quick and semi-witty "survival sarcasm." I usually respond with "If I had to walk around all day in your situation, all ignorant and missing the point of life, I might have to take my own life as well."

I know it sounds harsh. I know what they said is not exactly what they meant. Heaven knows how many times I have spoken before I considered my words and didn't choose to use them in the most logical and compassionate manner. But for them to make a cursory judgment about me and then proceed to string that phrase together demonstrates a lack of understanding about what my life entails and what is important to me.

The scariest part is that there are probably several people who actually meant it.

When people say things like this to me that I construe as hurtful or misguided, it is hard for me to not believe that their words demonstrate a fundamental lack of understanding about the person I am. I'm still amazed at how little we know about people until we take the time to reach out, connect, and find out what they do for a living, what they do for fun, and what their passions are.

When meeting me for the first time, people often try to make determinations about the quality of my life based on what they think my life would be like if they were to live it. Sadly, though, based on what they say to me and how they react to my situ-ation, most people simply internalize the things they believe they wouldn't be able to do if they were disabled.

People still approach me every day and ask, "How can you be so happy living in a wheelchair and not having legs?"

All I can do is look into their eyes and explain, "It seems to me that my disability exists more in your mind than it does in mine."

I have what I consider to be a minimal physical disability. A large portion of the population also self-identify as people with disabilities. Many of them have far greater everyday challenges than mine. I just do not have a pair of normal functioning legs. But with the addition of a small manual wheelchair, I am practically able to function as an able-bodied person in most settings.

It really isn't true for me to say that I don't have any legs, because I do have very short femur bones attached to my pelvis. Doctors call them stumps. I call them little legs because they look much like regular legs except they just end early. As I have grown, they have gotten longer. As an adult, both of them are now about fifteen inches long, measured while sitting down, from the back of my rear to the base of my foot. There is no scarring or irregular tissue where the leg bones end, and my feet are at-tached on the tip of the femur. They look like a natural extension of my body because they are.

I have never been shamed by the physical, disabling characteristics of my body. And yet, I choose not to wear shorts that reveal the end of my legs and feet. I have found that the full reveal just causes longer and more direct stares. I don't really mind keeping myself covered; it allows me some degree of control over my world.

But I do have an exception to this rule. As a professional speaker and consultant, I have the pleasure of sharing my ideas with a variety of audiences. When I speak to children at their school, they always want to know if I have feet. If I am wearing longer open-ended shorts during an event, I'll show my feet to the kids. It is a great moment, because everyone gives me their full attention. I tell them, "My feet don't look like your feet. But they're *my* feet, so I like them!"

I always present my right foot first; it has a bit more of a heel than the left one. If you look at it from the top down (my angle), it looks like a closed fist with a single index finger/toe extended on top with a toenail. When I was in college, I wore a large silver toe ring on it. Not many people saw it, but a cool able-bodied friend of mine had one on his big toe. I saw his and, well, you can guess the rest.

Some skin on the side looks like it is folding into itself, creating a small cavern. When I show the children, I tell them, "I am not sure why it is there; it's just my foot's belly button."

I think my left foot looks like the top of a duck's head. It has a heel on the left side and then it triangulates into the foundation of a toe. The base of the toe extends out and bends down like the tip of a regular toe. I sometimes share this story with the young students: When I was a child. I painted it to look like a duck's head and then performed a funny pup-pet routine on long family road trips for my sister in the back of our car. I have always found humor to be helpful tool to connect with people.

In my childhood, the first way I got around was in my parents' arms. I was held and carried much of the time like a sack of potatoes or an oversized bag of groceries. My mother likes to describe it more as a tender hand on my bottom and her arm sup-porting my back. When I wasn't being held, I could crawl. But it was more of a scoot, sliding around by moving my arms and pulling on furniture, walls, and people.

As I got older, when I could sit up, I would use my arms to move around. I could balance myself pretty well because, although I didn't have regular-length legs, my little legs were long enough to brace myself.

My mom called the way I moved on the floor a bunny hop. She is the only one I allow to call it that because I'm not totally comfortable with the name. It sounded silly and every time she said it, all I could think about was the Easter Bunny hopping around, delivering eggs.

I do have to admit, it does look like the way a rabbit moves, especially when they lean forward and put out their front legs and then bring their back legs forward. In a sense, that is exactly what I did and still do to get around when I'm on the ground.

Next came a stroller, still being pushed and directed by my parents. However, my first form of self-propelled transportation was a white and red Tonka truck. I would pull myself up, lay on the trailer, and push the truck around with my arms. The thick black wheels would make a rumbling noise on our wooden floor as I drove around the dining room.

I would turn by gently hitting the cab of the truck with one arm and then propel-ling it forward with the other. The best parts of driving were the highways I would blaze in the deep green shag carpet in our living room.

Luckily, my grandfather was gifted in his ability to modify my toys, so I could play with them. I enjoyed the addition of levers on metal pedal cars and a special hand-crafted custom tricycle that I powered by using my arms and hands instead of legs and feet.

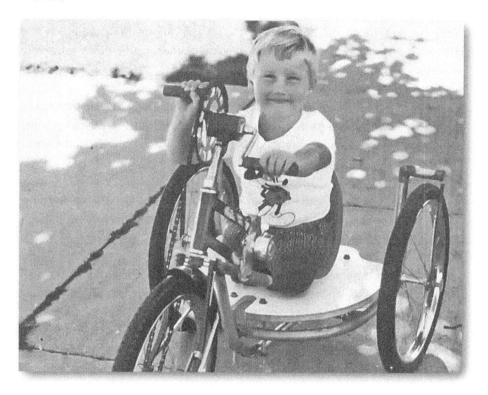

My family explored different ideas for how I could deal with the stairs in our home. Early on, my father recognized my ability to use physical strength to maneuver my body in different ways. He realized that all he needed to do was install the pull handles from a regular set of drawers into the side wall of the staircase. With those additions, I could grab the handles and pull myself up and down the stairs while doing a modi-fied shoulder roll. As I got bigger and stronger, I could lift my body completely with my arms and balance on each step with my torso. This provided me with the initial strength to know that if I had to get somewhere, I could do it myself. I didn't have to rely on someone to take care of my most basic needs.

As I grew, my journey of learning how to "walk" took me down the road of using a variety of devices that got me off the ground in numerous ways. Some were as simple as a modified bucket with wheels, some as complicated as a custom molded seating sys-tem with legs and spring-powered feet. The latter was called a Toronto Walker. I would propel myself forward by leaning to one side, compressing the leg, taking the pressure off the opposite "foot," and swinging my body around to the other side. I always thought I must have looked like a penguin, slowly lumbering where I needed to go.

Upon reflection, the experts probably thought it would help develop my balance above the floor, train me to shift my weight to take individual steps, and give me more basic exercise. I didn't use it for very long. It was too cumbersome and I thought, *why can't I just get around on the floor myself ?*

My favorite form of everyday transportation back then was a small yellow skate-board. It was practical and easy. It gave me speed, independence, and range; I used it on the first day of preschool.

At the age of three, my parents enrolled me in a pre-kindergarten class at a school called La Prairie, which I later learned was a special school for kids with disabilities.

But again, I wasn't disabled—at least, I didn't think so. I did a ton of art projects and I enjoyed playing with the giant red ball while I rolled around on the ground. But I also remember this overall feeling of not really belonging with the other children who couldn't speak, wouldn't play with me, and didn't move on their own. I didn't feel "disabled" like them. I was just me.

I talked to my parents, telling them I just didn't feel like I fit in. They listened and, when it was time, my parents enrolled me in half-day kindergarten class. It was located by our house at the "normal" public elementary school where my sister would be in the first grade.

Kindergarten was great! I was able to attend school with my friends from the neighborhood, having the same experiences they did. My friends accepted me as I was, and I saw myself as just one of them. Nothing special. Sure, I did things a bit differently, but in my mind, I could do anything they could do...and I did everything they did.

Little did I know that one of my differences which allowed me to ride a skateboard in kindergarten would make me the *coolest* kid in the class. At the time, there were no speed limits in the hallways. Of course later, that all changed. I guess all rules are in place because someone abuses a privilege.

All the other students wanted to know why they couldn't ride their skateboards in the hallways like I could. My teacher told them I could do it because I was special: I didn't have legs. I guess the other students didn't really see me as that different after all.

I was granted the extra ability to ride anywhere I wanted to for good reasons. It kept me from getting my pants dirty. It allowed me to put things on the front of the skateboard to carry them. I could go as fast as everyone else when they walked. More importantly, I saw the rules changed for me, and it made me feel special.

I did not view myself as being challenged in the way others may have seen me. My disability allowed me to be unique. I was different, and at that age, being different was pretty cool.

CHAPTER 2

The Virtue of Walking

During my early years of attending school, my doctors were constantly trying to explain to my parents the virtues of me being able to walk instead of using the skateboard. The professionals believed that at some point I would want to walk with artificial legs to have a more "normal" life. They believed it would be easier for me to "fit in" and that I would not be stared at by people. They felt it was important for me to start on that path as quickly as possible.

Although wheelchairs were available, the option was never seriously considered for me at that time. The wheelchairs in the late '70s were very heavy, even in smaller sizes. Weighing at least fifty pounds, they were difficult to manage. By using one, I would become dependent on other people to lift the chair in and out of cars and make my mobility far more complicated. Using a wheelchair then was nothing like using one now.

In the 1980s, due to steps, narrow doorways, and the absence of curb cuts, very few places were accessible for wheelchair users. There was no way I could use it in my family home because of the stairs. Finally, the concept of me using a wheelchair was dismissed because it didn't contribute to that larger goal of my being up and walking. A wheelchair would have been a step back from everyone else's goals.

Another idea the medical professionals considered was cutting off my feet to make the artificial legs work better. I had never considered amputating a part of my body. That's just what it was—my body, part of me. I didn't think there was anything wrong with it. Even though I was only six years old, I remember how their suggestion bothered me deeply, because I didn't want to permanently remove parts of my body to accomplish something I wasn't sure I would be able to do anyway. I had a lot weighing on my mind—big decisions to make. Was there really that much wrong with me, that doctors wanted to amputate a part of me?

POINT TO PONDER: Imagine if you were in my position. How would you have felt?

Eventually, the doctors did change their minds and I got to keep my feet. They said my foot with the toe might be able to trigger motion in the false legs sometime in the future, so it would be all right if I kept them. But that didn't prevent me from having horrific nightmares for years about the doctors coming in and amputating my feet while I slept.

With the doctors' suggestions, I was forced to try false legs and wear them in school. I hated those legs. When I tried to walk with them, the suction wouldn't stay sealed, and the prosthetics would eventually fall off. This forced the first major design change for the prosthesis.

The new legs were made of wood and plastic with the open areas made to fit my legs perfectly from molds they made. A metal hinge on each side connected them to a leather belt around my waist. As I was tied into the belt, my waist and hips carried the legs and controlled my balance. The area outside of my groin rested on the top edges of the hollow oak legs to carry my weight as my little legs slipped inside the holes crafted for them. This made all standing and movement painful and difficult. I had poor balance, and a pair of crutches was added for stability. I became a four-point walker.

Instead of developing a walking gait with each individual leg, the best possibility was to bring both legs forward at the same time. The doctors called how I walked "swinging through" with the legs. They came to the name specifically because that is how it looked. I would lean forward, plant both crutches a few feet out in front of me, then lift myself up and support my weight on the crutches while swinging the legs out in front of me. As the forward momentum of my body weight came over the top of the legs, I had to put forward pressure on the hinge in the knee with my little leg to keep it from buckling and causing me to fall.

It always appeared that I was leaning forward with bad posture. I didn't have bad posture; I just didn't want to fall on my face or bottom.

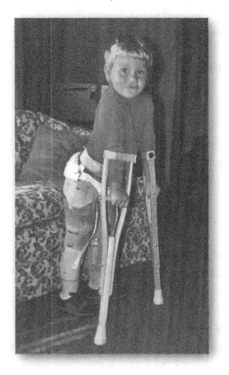

I just couldn't see how this could work. In essence, my doctors tied thirty pounds of dead weight to my body and it made me tired. They made me utilize wood crutches in my hands, which kept me from carrying anything. The uneasiness of the balancing act of the legs and knees brought uncertainty to my every step. It was unrealistic, and much more difficult for me to get around than the "natural" way—on a skateboard.

I would alternate between the two forms of mobility, even though using the legs instead of the skateboard was no easy task. For the first time, I started to feel truly "disabled" by the equipment designed to help me. When I used the skateboard, I was independent. I could carry everything on the front of the board and go as fast as ev-eryone else. I didn't feel different. This was just me.

The doctors kept recommending I continue using prosthetic legs, and in the third grade, my parents decided that I should wear the legs full time in school. I know that my parents truly wanted to do the right thing for me. They thought that by having me walk with legs in school, it would prepare me for using them the rest of my life. My parents wanted the best for me, and I trusted them. However, my real problems started when I lost all ability to take care of myself because I had to walk on those legs. It took all my concentration and effort just to stay upright. Sometimes, I would fall in the school hallways when they got too crowded. In short, it was difficult.

My friends were constantly pressed into service to carry my books and my lunch and to write the homework instructions down for me at the end of class, because I had to leave early to get a head start to my next class. The first few times, they would do it out of courtesy and friendship. Eventually, though, it became a job, and they started to distance themselves from me. It wasn't until twenty years later, when I saw one of them at a grocery store, that the hurtful truth came out. I asked, "Hey, I know it was a really long time ago, but I was wondering if you remembered why we stopped being friends in elementary school?"

He paused, then replied, "You know, I still feel bad about what happened. We all got really tired of helping you all the time, so we just decided to stop being your friend." Think of the weight of that revelation. Those thirty-pound legs were tooth-picks in comparison.

POINT TO PONDER: Have you ever been abandoned at a time you needed help the most? Have you ever left someone behind? How did it make you feel?

All this time, I had thought I'd done something that had betrayed them as a friend. I never considered that my legs had anything to do with it.

I became isolated at school; a few teachers felt sorry for me and regularly helped me when they could. One of my gym teachers noticed this happening and offered a solution that was supposed to make my life easier. Instead of asking other students to help me carry my books, she recommended that I wear a backpack so I could carry them myself. I think she was on the right track with her solution, but it forced me to trek all the way back to my locker after each class. I was only strong enough to carry one class' worth of books and folders in addition to the legs and crutches at a time. Balancing was extremely challenging, but I did it.

I think everyone's childhood and early adolescence is difficult. It's a time when we're trying to figure out who we're going to be. But my childhood coupled these issues with trying to figure out how I'd be getting around for my entire life. My parents did their best to shield me from feeling this way. And I often worried that they missed out on being able to share certain things with me because I didn't have legs. Yet, as a family, we found a great many new things to do together. My mother told me she never felt like my disability had ever held our family back from doing things we all wanted to do.

Thanks Mom.

CHAPTER 3

Faith Healer

When I was in the fifth grade, my mother broke down to peer pressure from some of her friends and people in the community and took me to a faith healer. I'll give you a moment to digest that... A faith healer.

Needless to say, I did not want to go. I never had legs, and I got around fine on my skateboard. I was finally getting used to using the prosthetics in school, even though I didn't like it.

I traveled with my mom from our home to a church called the Shalom Faith Center in Madison, Wisconsin. I was told I was to meet with a woman at the end of a church service who claimed to be a faith healer.

As you can imagine, it was a long night. All the people she was going to heal had to sit up front and listen to her preach for what seemed like an eternity.

When it came time to start the healings, she took what I determined were the easy ones first. There were people who were suffering from hidden disabilities, things that weren't apparent visually. She laid hands on a few with high blood pressure and some with headaches. There was a person with severe diabetes, who claimed it caused her partial blindness.

The faith healer put her hands on the woman's head and massaged her face and eye sockets for a few minutes, all the while leading the people in the church in prayer. We watched as the person with diabetes testified to the congregation that she could now actually see better than before. It was scripted and staged as if the presence of the all-loving and immortal God had saved her sight.

I was meant to be the healer's finale, the big finish to the show. I did not fully understand the magnitude of what was about to take place, but there was nothing comforting or loving about any of it. She reached out to bring me to the front of the stage, while moving around maniacally and speaking in tongues.

I started feeling self-conscious, and it upset me. I declined her invitation to go up on stage and glanced at my mom. She looked at me, told the healer "No," and the woman moved away.

The faith healer asked everyone in the congregation to pray for me to grow legs and escape the obvious nightmare I was living. After trying to channel all the love from the almighty God and the power he brings, she had to give up on saving me and making me "whole." She told everyone that God spoke to her, and the absence of legs was entirely my fault.

My fault!

The faith healer professed to everyone in the church that I "did not have enough faith in God."

I was ten.

I did not believe I needed "fixing."

My mom gripped my hand and pulled me into a hug. As we were leaving the church, people approached me and said everything was going to be fine. I still didn't really understand what this lady's show was supposed to be all about. I just felt weird about the whole thing.

On the way home, my mom did the best she could to make the situation better. Over a dish of ice cream at Baskin Robbins, she said, "It's not your fault."

I looked up at her with an expression that conveyed that I already knew that.

"God doesn't work that way," she went on, "and I'm really sorry I made you go through all of that. You'll never have to do anything like that again if you don't want to."

This episode really made me think about my situation in a completely different way than I had ever before. What if I had shown up at school the next day with real legs given to me by an all-accepting and loving God who fixed something he overlooked when I was conceived? How would I explain that to other fifth graders? I was relieved that nothing happened, so I would not have to explain it to my friends. Today, as I look back, I realize that real emotional and spiritual damage could have been done, shifting my mindset from a can-do attitude to one of winners and losers based on who God decides he wants to help.

Life continued on as normal, prosthetics and all. I hated them every day. One day at school, I was walking past the gym teacher's office with my legs and crutches when I happened to see the school's wheelchair in the office. It was the standard type of wheelchair with leg rests, handles, and metal armor on the sides, completely unlike the one I use today.

I stopped and poked my head in. There wasn't anyone in the office.

Boldly, I went in, unfolded the wheelchair, and sat down in it with my legs on. We were a match. I immediately leaned back and put it into a "wheelie." I rode around in it for a couple of minutes and realized I didn't need the crutches anymore. I put them in the corner. Then, I also realized I didn't need to wear the legs to push it around. I unbuckled the belt, slid the prosthetics off my little legs, and left them in the corner, too. Imagine my relief and newfound freedom.

For the rest of the day, I used the wheelchair until my mom came to get me. The other students got out of my way in the hallway and the teachers started moving chairs in the classrooms to make space for the wheelchair. No one asked me why I was using the chair; it just seemed like it was "normal."

Just before my mom came to pick me up, I went back to the office, put the legs on, and grabbed the crutches and walked out to the car. It was perfect, in the sense that she always told me I had to wear the legs to school, but she never said anything about having to actually wear them during the day.

The next day, I went to school with the legs on, and as soon as my mom drove away, I went to that same gym office to get the wheelchair. I took off my legs and used the wheelchair all day until my mom came and picked me up. My plan worked again.

I repeated this process every day for two weeks. The final day of my freedom came when, by accident, I had forgotten my lunch. Mom came to school to bring the lunch, she came to class to see me and saw me using the wheelchair.

A stern expression came over her face. Later that afternoon, she let loose. "All of the things we had been working toward, all the things the experts have told us you need to do to be normal and have all of your options open for the future are at risk by you taking the easy way out, and not using the legs!"

My parents informed all of my teachers that I was to wear the legs at all times. I was being watched at school and at home—I had to wear the legs when I was out in public. I didn't want to wear them, but I did. I wore them because as a kid, I did what I was told to do by my parents. They were supposed to know what was good for me. But how many parents get to take the class that teaches them the right things to do for their child with a unique disability?

Back then, it was a different time. My father told me about being asked if he wanted to baptize me *afterrr* the Sunday service at church, so as to not draw attention to the fact that my parents had a disabled child. Many families with children who had disabilities would just keep their children at home out of sight. It was easier for families, physically and emotionally, to keep people hidden away, rather than trying to make a life for someone whom everyone thought would never be able to negotiate the world on their own. My parents and doctors encouraged me to wear the legs in public to appear as "normal" as possible.

Such is not the case today, thankfully, although sometimes members of the general public still congratulate me for functioning by myself and being out in the world. Gee—you're welcome, I guess.

I am not mad at my parents for wanting the best for me according to cultural and social norms. They thought they were helping me. But when I was a child, I just didn't have the words or emotional wherewithal to explain to my parents what I was experi-encing. The best way I can explain it now is by saying that I was looking for the freedom to be me in my natural form and gain acceptance for who I was, not who other people thought I needed to be.

POINT TO PONDER: Have you ever felt like you were different from others? Was this difference out of your control? How did it make you feel?

At that time, I wish I had a track record of success to show my parents how I thought I could succeed at school while using the wheelchair. It not only gave me a different kind of freedom of mobility, but also a confidence of stature. The wheelchair allowed me to have a conversation with someone and not have to worry about falling down at any time for no apparent reason. I could move along with my friends and continue talking at the same time. And, most importantly, I didn't have physical weights tied to my body, making everything I wanted to do so much harder.

When I was in school, I believe I intrinsically knew how to accept myself, relax, and live the life I wanted. Scooting, crawling, skateboarding, and wheeling around with every conceivable wheeled vehicle became my convenience for experiencing life to the fullest. That was me, and that was the way I did things. I wish other people had accepted that then, too, the way they do today.

Maybe I should have tried to be more adamant about using a wheelchair or the skateboard instead of the prosthetics. Now I realize what they thought was best for me wasn't best because I was already "complete."

If you know someone who is experiencing life in their own way, listen to them. Allow them to live how they want, using the methods that work best for them.

They are probably becoming quite the expert on their situation and may well know what's right, comfortable, and "better" for them.

POINT TO PONDER: When in your life have others tried to impose on you what they think is best for you, and were they right or wrong? Have you ever caught yourself being one of those "others"? Hopefully, you remember to give them the chance to surprise you.

CHAPTER 4
Getting Around on New Legs

The first few generations of my prosthesis had no air holes in the leg to release the moisture and sweat that accumulated at the bottom of the leg while I walked in it. Each time I went to the bathroom, I dumped out the pools of sweat inside each prosthetic.

My grandfather cut out air holes in the sides of the legs. The doctors were angry with us because they thought we were "compromising the integrity" of the prosthetics, but we were just making them more comfortable by letting my little legs breathe inside them. When we were at our doctor appointments, other families with children who had prostheses would see the holes in the side of my legs and ask about them. After our explanation of why we did it, sure enough, when we would see the families again, their children would have holes in their legs as well. Eventually, the doc-tors started cutting air holes in other children's prosthetic legs.

Every couple of years, a new pair of legs was made for me. Their evolution from being exclusively formed from wood to a mixture of wood with plastic resins made the legs a little better and a little lighter each time. And as I grew, I needed more mate-rial for the legs to "grow" proportionally with me. There was never a time I realized a weight savings. They always felt heavy to me.

The only good thing about getting new legs was that each time, I was able to decide how tall I wanted to be. I would always find out the height of my best friend, and I would go a half-inch taller. But then, he would keep growing, too.

Architecturally speaking, transitioning to a four-story middle school from an elementary school that was all on one level was my next challenge. Thank goodness it had an elevator.

However, all the school's entrances had at least seven stairs I would have to climb to get in, so the custodians let my parents drive our car down a service ramp into the basement and boiler room of the school. It smelled like fuel oil and garbage, but it was like being able to get into school through the Bat Cave. During those snowy Wisconsin winters, I never had to worry because I would get in my parents' car in our garage and get out at school inside of the cave. My only disappointment was I never did see Bruce Wayne, Batman, Robin, or Alfred.

The thing I loved most in middle school was music. And yet, the choir section of the building was in a new addition, without elevator access. To get to the classroom, it was a twelve-stair climb down with my legs and crutches, out of the main building, and a split section of four and three steps. I hated all those steps, but I loved singing in the choir.

This building was also my first daily introduction to highly dangerous Terrazzo floors, the ultimate in slippery hazards for people with canes and crutches. The floor was truly an amazing invention—so smooth, so flat, just the perfect way to literally break a new pair of legs, crutches, and maybe an arm at the beginning of the school year. The school took all summer to clean and polish the surface. I always feared the extended breaks from school when they would put all the polishing work in on the floors.

As part of advancing to the new school, the doctors encouraged me to wear the legs not only all day there, but also when I was out in public. This was meant to train me to be as independent as possible.

At this same time, my mother insisted that my sister and I take piano lessons to help foster our interest in music. It was something she valued from her childhood. The only challenge was that the piano teacher lived downtown on the second floor above a business storefront in a building without an elevator. This meant that after school each Wednesday, I wore my legs to the twenty-two-step staircase I had to climb with my prosthesis to get to my piano lesson.

I would back up against the hardwood stairs with my heels against the bottom of the first step. The doctors always told me to face away from looking at the stairs while climbing them, because I would have a better chance catching myself if I fell forward down the stairs instead of falling backward and just breaking my neck.

I grabbed the railing with one hand and gripped the handle of my crutch with the other. I had to push up on both the railing and the crutch to lift myself to get to the next stair. The motion was tricky—not only was I trying to move vertically, but I needed to move myself backward after hoping I had gone up far enough to clear the front lip of the next stair behind me.

I was really just guessing each time to see if I was going to make it, because I couldn't see what I was doing. Step after step, I repeated the process until I reached the top of the landing or fell face forward back down all the steps I had just climbed.

To go back down, I would simply reverse the process facing away from the stairs. I also had to carry my other crutch hand while I was navigating the steps, because I couldn't exactly leave a crutch at the bottom when I would need it at the top.

I never got good at climbing all those stairs or playing the piano. Every part of taking my piano lessons was an adventure: I would fall on the stairs on the way up, on the way down, and I could barely sight read the piano music. Beethoven could rest easy—I posed no threat.

After attending three years of middle school with the slippery floors and all the stairs in my life, I learned that all of the "fall training" I went through at the hospital was worth it. Yes, "fall training." When I was learning to use fake legs, they taught me how to fall forward in the best way. On my way to the floor, the specialists recommended releasing the crutches quickly by throwing them so I could catch myself with my hands. If I should happen to fall backward, I was instructed to tuck my head against my chest to protect it, because there would be no good way to catch myself or brace my fall.

This training also consisted of getting pushed down, or having my crutch slip out from under me on a floor coated with wax. Then, I was told to try many ways of getting up (which often involved falling down again).

What I have learned throughout my childhood is that falling is bad, no matter who you are. This is especially terrible for a person on prosthetics, whether it happens by accident or on purpose. It is scary for everyone involved. Then, I had a life-changing realization.

I was about to enter high school, and I was tired of the prosthetics. I had given them a solid try in middle school. At some point, how I got around was going to have to be *my* decision. There was going to be a time when I would finally have enough credibility and courage to make my own decisions.

I was tired of the accommodations others pressed on me, especially those that did not work. They didn't have the desired effect of making my life easier; in fact, many times these accommodations made life more difficult.

I decided to play a trick on my parents. When in public with my family, I started falling down on purpose to illustrate how poorly the legs were working out for me.

As I fell or "accidentally" tripped, everyone around me would gasp, look horri-fied, and run over to help me. When I fell strategically at the grocery store, I would be standing in the checkout line with the other shoppers. Then, for no apparent reason, I would fall to the floor while throwing my crutches sideways into the racks of candy.

Everyone would look on with horror in their eyes, and I would be crying on the floor and acting as if I was pain.

They would all look at my mother and say things like, "That doesn't look like that works very well for him." Or "It looks like he's getting hurt!"

It was perfect.

During the fall, I learned to throw my crutches into other items to amplify the noise. I knew how to release the knees to make the wood sound like it was cracking. The only problem I ran into was with how the top of the legs met my groin area.

My fake falls always backfired a little. I was growing as a man, and each time I fell, the impact from the top of the legs smashing together would pinch my privates—*hard.* It was excruciating, but I was willing to expose myself to that short-term pain to illustrate the long-term pain I was going to be in if I had to wear the legs for the rest of my life.

While I was hurt and bruised, my mom wanted to find a quick solution because she really wanted grandchildren. I brought up the idea of the wheelchair again, and we started exploring it seriously as a primary method of locomotion.

Accessibility-wise, it was the right time. I was about to transition from middle school to high school. That meant a new building and new accessibility opportunities. The new high school I would attend was all on one level. It was perfect for a wheelchair user.

My parents started coming around to my way of thinking about not using the legs. However, my doctor still felt that I could blend in better with the new high school students if I used the prosthetics. He even thought that if I wanted to use a wheelchair, I should have my false legs hanging off the front of the chair to make me look a little bit less conspicuous.

At the beginning of my freshman year in high school, my father and I went to the Shriner's Hospital for children in Chicago. That would be my last appointment for using prosthetics. My father told me that this was going to be a really big decision... and it would be mine. Furthermore, I would have to explain my decision to the doctor.

The doctor came into the room, my file in hand, and he immediately inquired about the amount of time I was wearing the legs and how they were working. I had that feeling you get in your stomach when you know you are about to disappoint someone.

I explained to the doctor that I wasn't wearing the legs because they still weren't comfortable, and I didn't feel good wearing them. I told him that I believed that I wasn't ever going to want to wear them again. He asked me if I was sure, because this was going to be a large decision in a few different ways.

First, I would be going in a direction that he didn't see many people go due to the public pressure that was directed toward people who are different—people who choose to live their lives in a way that is out of the ordinary.

"Your life is going to be much harder if you choose not to learn how to walk," the doctor told me. Even today, I remember how serious his face was.

He said that many of his patients who were missing body parts who chose not to use mobility prostheses still had cosmetic ones hanging off their bodies or mounted to a wheelchair just to save them from the added attention they would get from not look-ing "normal."

"It doesn't matter to me," I said. In fact, I could not imagine hanging something off the front of my wheelchair just to alleviate someone else's concerns.

The doctor sighed heavily. "If you reject this next pair of legs from the Shriner's organization," he began, "you will not have the opportunity to change your mind—the cost of the legs will not be covered by them."

All of my future artificial legs would have to be purchased by my family.

I looked over at my dad. The value of each of the pairs of legs I had been receiving from Shriner's was in the thousands of dollars, and we didn't have insurance for that. This was the moment of decision. It was legs or no legs, for the rest of my life.

But I knew. I was sure I would never want prosthetic legs again.

After rendering my decision, the doctor stated, "By choosing a wheelchair as your primary means of transportation, you're deciding to have a harder life, especially because of all the physical accessibility limitations you'll run into every day."

That was fine. It was easier for me to get out of a wheelchair and climb stairs car-rying the wheelchair than it was for me to climb up stairs with the prosthetic legs.

I left the hospital feeling as if a weight had been lifted off me. I was now moving on to a new chapter in my life: using a wheelchair full time. I was getting back to what I considered "normal." It was those prosthetic "legs" that were actually keeping me disabled.

CHAPTER 5
Disability Drawbacks

A s I was exploring my newfound freedom with my wheelchair, I wanted to go places and do things I never thought I could while wearing the legs. I applied and was accepted to participate in the famous Space Camp in Huntsville, Alabama. Pardon the pun, but I was over the moon with excitement when my parents told me the news. And then, we alerted them of my disability. They canceled my invi-tation because they thought I wouldn't be able to do all the experiments and fit into all the simulators.

Houston, we had a problem.

There was no mechanism or process in place to make them reconsider or even think about admitting me, a kid with a disability. That was the last time we told any-one in charge of anything about my disability until we arrived. My family learned the rule, "It is easier to ask for forgiveness than to seek permission."

POINT TO PONDER: What do you think of my family's philosophy on choosing not to tell organizations or events about my disability until we showed up? Would you have done the same thing?

Utilizing our new rule, I *was* allowed to participate at Badger Boys State Leadership Camp. My school advisor left quickly after dropping me off, and there was no one willing to make the two-hour drive to take me back home. I also prom-ised the camp officials that I wouldn't need any help. They didn't offer any either, so, I stayed.

There were still accessibility challenges I faced when deciding to use the wheel-chair over the prosthetics. Badger Boys Camp was held at a private college with stairs I had to hand climb. Some of my new friends carried my wheelchair to help me get into the dining hall, my dorm room, and the group shower area. I couldn't bring my wheelchair into the bathroom because the door wasn't wide enough to fit it through.

Each morning I would wear my bathing suit into the bathroom area, get com-pletely undressed, and sit naked on the group shower room floor. I dragged my lower half toward the row of shower heads, trying to find an open one. All through everyone else's dirty, soapy water, I tried to get clean alongside everyone else.

I was glad that I attended the camp, but it was then when I realized there was go-ing to be a whole new set of challenges to navigate if I was going to use my wheelchair full time. It was quite clear—the world still wasn't made for me, or anyone who needed accessibility options.

Mobility-wise, I was very independent in high school. By using a wheelchair and freeing myself from the prosthetics, I felt more normal around other people than I had ever felt before. I became more interested in trying new things because I thought I could do them.

I was given a locker at the end of a row so I could use it when other students were at theirs, too. The teachers let me use a faculty restroom because the regular boys' and girls' bathrooms weren't accessible. Most, not all, of the school was accessible. And yet, I was beginning to learn that this wasn't the case with the rest of the real world.

On my sixteenth birthday, my family passed down to me our brown Chrysler minivan with wood grain panels on the sides. I had taken driver's education as a soph-omore because the teacher had a set of hand controls left over from a disabled family member who wasn't driving anymore. He installed them on the school's training car, and I proficiently passed the class and my driver's test.

The minivan gave me the ability to get around—true independence. I found it to be a great leveling force. Now when people would go somewhere, I could go too and take them with me. I was able to help other people get around. The maintenance people at school even purchased and installed a handicapped parking sign in the student lot for me.

I started taking my newfound access for granted. I felt normal, no different than anyone else. I was a teenager who drove and went to high school; I had a normal life. And just as my classmates started to pursue the opposite sex, I too found an interest in them. I didn't think my difference should have an impact on starting a romantic relationship. I thought everyone would accept me. *Why should the fact that I don't have legs impact the person I am attracted to, since it doesn't affect me?e?e?* I didn't see my handicap as being a big deal, because to me, it wasn't.

I now know that my disability has a very real impact on my friends, and on strangers. The consequences of my disability on the people I am in relationships with are real. In terms of romantic relationships, the first time I learned about this was the hard way. It occurred when I asked my first real girlfriend to the homecoming dance, the fall term of my junior year of high school.

Jenny and I met the summer before my junior year. We would go to each other's houses and watch movies together. Love, right?

I had always heard about school dances, seen them on television and in movies. I loved music and wanted to have the chance to be around other people dancing, feeling the music. I knew that if I had any chance of having a complete high school experience, I needed to attend a school dance.

Even though Jenny was my first girlfriend, I was feeling relatively confident that she would say yes if I asked her to go. Yet, there was still this uneasy nervousness about asking her to the dance. *What if she said no?* I'd be crushed.

I put up a brave front and asked Jenny. When she responded with a "Yes," it was one of my proudest moments. I was now on my way to achieving a full high school experience.

I was so excited to pick her up at her house. Our parents took an annoying amount of pictures. But I didn't let it bother me—I had the entire night left with Jenny. After the pictures were finally over, we went out to dinner and then to the dance. As soon as we entered the building, she said that she had to go to the ladies' room.

Five minutes passed, then ten. It was now going on fifteen minutes and still no Jenny. I was starting to get worried. Did she get sick from something she ate? I saw my friend Kim standing with a few other people, so I asked if she would mind running a recon mission for me.

Kim returned from the restricted area only a few minutes later and I noticed something was wrong. Upset, she approached me and said, "Jenny says she's really sorry, but she won't come out." I had to coax out of Kim what she said next.

She said Jenny told her, "I have no idea how to dance with Matt. I don't know why he would have even asked me to the dance 'cause he wouldn't be able to do it." According to Kim, Jenny said, "I just feel really uncomfortable being out in such a public place with him. I wish he would just go home."

I didn't want to show Kim how upset I was. I just thanked her and told her I appreciated her telling me the truth.

All the excitement of the night was dead. All the visions of what I thought it would be like to be at a dance with my girlfriend exploded into a million pieces, shattering in front of my face.

Crowded thoughts pounded my brain. *Why didn't Jenny say something to me? Were there other things she couldn't tell me too?*

And of course, I wondered, *did Jenny even like me at all?*

The haunting thought then entered my head: *Is this going to be something I am going to have to deal with forever when I am in relationships with people?*

That scared me.

I grew mad, embarrassed, and uncomfortable all at the same time. I no longer had a date or a friend to go with to the dance. My ignorant teenage mindset had prepared me to achieve a new rung on the ladder of fulfillment in high school. And now, it was all taken away by the one girl in my life who I thought loved me—naively, because she had agreed to go to the dance with me.

I had no idea that I could be rejected for something I didn't see myself: the absence of my legs. I thought Jenny had accepted me for the person I was, but instead, I was cast off because of something that was out of my control.

All I could do was sit on the side of the dance floor and look at all the other couples having a great time. It felt like they were mocking me as I sat there alone. For the first time, I wondered if anyone would ever want to be romantically involved with me because of my differences. I didn't know where to go from there.

Then I saw it: a large crowd of girls surrounding the DJ. They were all having a blast, begging and smiling and fighting to get his attention. He was doing his best to make them happy by playing the music they wanted to hear. He belonged there with them. I knew deep inside that I could belong if I could do his job.

I left the dance that night with a mission in my heart: I wanted to become a DJ. I did not realize that in high school, I already had more than half of what I needed to be a DJ. I already owned the twenty-three songs a DJ needed to play at the school dance. I just needed the other stuff. I left the dance and went back home to develop a plan to tell my dad.

When I arrived at home, my father met me at the door and asked why I was home so early. I explained the fiasco to him. He told me that there would be many other women out there who would love me for all the right reasons. On the outside, I acted like I agreed with what he was saying. But on the inside, I was rolling my eyes thinking, "*Sure, Dad.*"

It has taken me many years to get to a place where I don't blame Jenny and get angry for what she did that night. Now, I realize she was not emotionally prepared to handle her decision to go to the dance with me. It did not make her a bad person; it made her a person who wasn't prepared to handle a different relationship dynamic than she had had previously.

Until that night's dance, I had been sheltered from any consequence of being rejected by someone or judged by someone based on my disability. It wouldn't be my last experience like that.

Later on in high school, I made some poor choices socially and cheated with the girlfriend of one of my best friends. He had been one of the first people to help me with all the manual labor involved with setting up my DJ service. I lost a friend and the person who made it all possible for me to do that job. When he confronted me on the phone about it, he said, "If you weren't crippled, I'd come over there right now and kick your ass!"

It was the first time this friend had ever brought up the fact that I didn't have any legs. Before this, I assumed that he saw me for me and did not care about my disability. We were working together because we both enjoyed DJing. His statement introduced the idea that his interactions with me were still at least somewhat influenced by the fact he felt sorry for me because of my being disabled.

He would not give me the beating I obviously deserved because he perceived I was disabled—and I hated that. It made me feel even worse about what I had done. In my mind, it cheapened the friendship I had with him, even though I hadn't respected the relationship myself, having cheated with his girlfriend.

Just as Jenny had avoided me because I was disabled, I now understood that my best friend looked at me not as Matt, but as his friend with a disability. I was starting to realize that people were more focused on my disability than I was.

I didn't want people to perceive me as disabled, but they did anyway. Turning the tables on the situation, I eventually started to use this to my advantage—something I call "Disability Privilege."

PART 2
Disability Privilege

CHAPTER 1

College

t was the first day of college orientation, the next major step forward in my life. I was attending the University of Wisconsin – Whitewater campus. Both of my parents and my sister were alumni of the school. Within the university's mission statement was the directive to actively collaborate with students, faculty, and staff to create an inclusive, accessible university experience for people with a disability.

I was sitting in the auditorium with my parents, watching the student orientation leaders introduce campus life through skits and lectures. After the presentations, we were going to do a campus tour with the rest of the new students when a young woman named Wendy from the Office of Disability Student Services greeted us.

She directed us to her office on campus. I was impressed with all the special study spaces outfitted with the latest technology readers and translation machines designed to assist students with disabilities to achieve success in school.

After our office visit, Wendy gave my family our own tour of campus, point-ing out the visible accommodations, including Lee Hall. The first floor of the integrated four-story dormitory was the only completely accessible housing. I was to live there with all the other disabled men arriving on campus that semester. The building did have an installed elevator, which allowed me to make friends with other guys on other levels, but the only floor with accessible bathrooms was the first floor.

Out of a dozen residence halls on campus, only three had elevators. I found that to be a bit limiting when trying to meet and make friends. So, I just invited the people I wanted to be friends with to come over to my dorm, and it seemed to be fine.

Everyone in the office wanted to help welcome me. My parents and I were ushered into a special office of one of the administrators. She started asking very personal and specific questions about my life and my abilities. She asked about my personal financial resources, if I had normal bathroom capabilities, and if I could transfer on and off my bed. I answered everything as honestly as I could; my comments to her reflected my expectation that I could manage myself on campus and I didn't really need any help.

She put down her clipboard that had a long checklist of available services. She drew in a long breath and shook her head sideways as if she was saying no. I took it as her thinking that I wasn't a credible person to make my own decisions about what campus was going to be like for me. Although I know she didn't mean any disrespect, I couldn't help but feel it.

"College is an entirely new experience," she said. "There's no way for you to re-ally know what you need here." She listed all the special services the campus could provide a person with a disability. I could have note-takers attend class with me to take my notes. When there was a test I needed to complete, it could be administered in the Disabled Student Services Office, where someone would help me with it. I was allowed to select any class at any time without the worry of it being full. Apparently, the university assumed it must have been harder for me to get ready in the morning. Many other services were available too: People could even be assigned to do my laun-dry, clean my room, and help me with my daily activities. I could use a free accessible van service to ride to my classes or to go around town. The campus prioritized people with a disability having full access to all aspects of college, including having a rich social life.

"Back up," I said, trying to keep from laughing. Did I look helpless? "I have my own vehicle on campus, and I'm not planning on drinking or partying, so I don't think I'll need that."

Finished with her list, she looked at me, rolled her chair away from her desk, sighed, and declared, "Well, I guess we might be done here."

I felt like I had hurt her feelings. "I'm sorry," I said. "I really appreciate all the things you're willing to provide..." I trailed off, aware that my words weren't getting anywhere. I would be all right doing things by myself. I believe she really wanted to help, and I had kept her from doing what she thought was her job.

The fully-inclusive infrastructure the campus had created could really offset the challenges many students faced, both as they transitioned to college, and as they left their protected family situations at home. This was not my experience. I only need-ed to utilize the physical accommodations the university had already made, not the specialized support services. Wendy didn't realize this, and I can't blame her.

Many new students with a disability need all of those things. However, the way the additional support services were offered to me didn't feel right. Their assumption was that I might not have needed them, but would have really appreciated them, once I was up and running as a student. After finally winning the war against the experts who thought I needed prosthetic legs, I wasn't about to slide into letting more experts tell me what they thought I needed.

I never did take the university up on any of the special assistance they offered. My choices to not take advantage of their offerings separated me from most of the people on campus with disabilities. The students who chose to use the services spent an incredible amount of time within the offices. It served as not only an accessible space for them, but also as a larger support group for people who liked to be with other people like themselves.

I took for granted my abilities to independently get around, take notes, and manage daily personal maintenance. My inherent privilege provided me the wherewithal to make my own accommodations when needed and manage the struggles of going to college in a more able-bodied way. I learned in school that the more things I could do by myself without support from other people, the more friends I would have. That is what I really wanted.

POINT TO PONDER: Can you understand my desire to want to be "normal," if only to have more friends? Have you ever felt that way?

Most of the first-year students with disabilities, myself included, arrived on campus pushing around manual wheelchairs or walking with crutches and braces. Some, like me, managed their own mobility and some did not. I felt a sense of camaraderie with others on our floor. We brushed our teeth and got ready in the community bathroom every morning. All of us ate in the dining halls with a wide variety of students. We took an active role in our education, by going to class. But after the first semester, I started noticing a change in their social behavior.

The students who were able to get around by themselves were still doing so. But instead of doing it manually, they started using electric carts and power wheelchairs. Their newfound ease of mobility reduced the amount of exercise they received. They started eating meals outside of the regular dining areas. They stopped socializing with the rest of the students. Many local restaurants would deliver food to their rooms. There was no need for them to leave their dorm rooms—and they didn't.

One of my friends stopped showering every day. He said he had a bad attendant who took too long helping him in the morning. There wasn't enough time to do his full routine of maintenance, so he wasn't able to get fully clean every day. Instead of finishing the rest of his care himself, he just let it go and figured they would get to it tomorrow, even though that wasn't always the case. Some of the single rooms in my dorm started to smell bad from their poor hygiene habits.

Other disabled classmates only attended classes when they wanted to, with no repercussions if they missed too many days. If they really didn't want to go, they could apply for a medical withdrawal grade and it wouldn't affect their grade point averages.

All of the unneeded accommodations intended to lift these people up actually held them back from being the person they could have been. I saw changes in their motivation levels, self-esteem, and hygiene. I could tell who had accepted all of the extra services offered by the office.

While in college and after I graduated, I started to see a large group of people with disabilities just staying there—not graduating or advancing toward a career even after six or seven years of studying. I asked a few of them about their plans after graduation, and they said they didn't really have any. They found the university to be the safest, most accommodating and accessible place they had ever been. If they graduated and moved to a different city, they thought they would lose everything they had: a social group, someplace to be, full housing, transportation, and meals. If, upon graduating and getting a job, their income was too much, they could possibly lose their government-funded financial support for their personal care attendants. There wasn't any better situation than what they had. To punctuate their argument, they would actually ask, "Why should we graduate?"

I named their situation "over-accommodation." It is a condition people sometimes find themselves in after having all of their needs and more met by other people working on their behalf. People have been known to stop looking to provide for themselves and start expecting things to be done for them and given to them.

I must admit that I periodically experience these feelings as well. I expect people to hold the door for me and sometimes give me things for free because of the absence of my legs.

Any amount of accommodation could be considered an over-accommodation. But shouldn't the idea be to make the person as functional as possible? We can learn to avoid accommodation apathy, as too much of a good thing can have an adverse effect.

Attending college is a challenge for everyone. If someone with a disability is making a go of it, the hardship of operating in any environment not completely accessible can be insurmountable. The special accommodations offered by the Disabled Student Services on campus at the time had the best intentions of offering support and solutions to assist people in their efforts to succeed. But the extra support offered—especially when it might not have been needed—didn't serve as a safety net to help students achieve success. Instead, it became the support that eliminated their need to do things for themselves.

POINT TO PONDER: Getting help is nice, but have you ever had someone try and help you too much? How did it make you feel?

CHAPTER 2

The Privilege of Having a Disability

Many people have disabilities in some way. I define a "disability" as the con-sequence of an impairment or other challenge, which may be physical, cognitive, mental, sensory, emotional, developmental, or some combination of these, that requires special accommodations for an individual to function or succeed in society. I find the absence of traditional legs on my body to be disabling. But for others, a disability may manifest in a deterioration of their senses, the development of a disease, or mobility challenges at different stages of life.

If a person is constantly looking for a reason not to achieve, not to contribute, or not to fulfill their personal responsibilities to themselves and society, "disability" can serve as a convenient pass for that person. Conversely, in some people's eyes, when a person overcomes their challenges and achieves his or her potential in the face of adversity, it reveals the kind of character they possess.

My disability presents challenges to me every day. However, I try to anticipate and prepare for them. That is how I have found it best to live. When people see me do what I normally do, they approach me and congratulate me for doing a great job with whatever I am trying to accomplish.

Have you ever been on a team that was cheered on in competition? Do you re-member how amazing it felt to be part of something bigger than yourself, and then be recognized for your individual contribution to the team's success? Now imagine if everywhere you went, strangers would come up to you and tell you how amazing you were just for being there.

The absence of my legs inspires people to convey those good feelings and accolades upon me every day, just from my presence out in public. I just do the same things that everyone else does, like shopping, and because of the approach I have to take, my disability provides automatic interest and sympathy from other people.

I look at it as the primary advantage I have because of something I have identified as "Disability Privilege."

Merriam-Webster defines the word *privilege* as "a right or benefit that is given to some people and not to others."

In her book *35 Dumb Things Well-Intentioned People Say*, Maura Cullen describes privilege as "access to resources based solely on a person's status as a member of an advantaged group."

I describe Disability Privilege as:

1. Access to an inherent right, advantage, or higher class of service granted to or enjoyed by people with a disability beyond what is commonly offered to the able-bodied population in the United States.
2. A privileged position: the sympathetic position a person with a disability enjoys in society based on a perception that their life is harder or they cannot accomplish as much as an able-bodied person.
3. Providing immunity, preference, or the benefit of the doubt to people with disabilities based on the presence of a disability.

I know I am turning the generally accepted understanding of the word "privilege" on its head by broadening its definition beyond a "group's" denial of access to parts of majority culture by claiming it has positive attributes as well. However, Disability Privilege is still oppressive, because the accrued benefits to people with disabilities from the larger able-bodied culture. It is also a direct result of the denial of a higher general expectation for what disabled persons can accomplish simply based on the presence of a disability.

The mere existence of my disability grants me access to Disability Privilege. It does not make up for all the things I can't do because of the absence of my legs. But it does provide me with a special opportunity not given to most people in chance or causal encounters. It gives me a chance to surprise them. In the past, I have had people refer to me as an amazing "super cripple"—simply for being able to carry my own plate back to a table at a buffet.

Unfortunately, not all of the benefits of Disability Privilege are granted evenly to all people with disabilities. Many times, people with hidden disabilities, such as Post Traumatic Stress, dyslexia, anxiety, or depression are completely denied access to Disability Privilege because able-bodied people might not even judge them as having a "real" disability.

During regular first-time interactions, people with hidden disabilities are often-times "outed" or forced to self-disclose a limitation or to redefine their ability to a stranger. As this occurs, it changes the expectation and opens up the possibility for the person with the hidden disability to be unable to accomplish many other things in the stranger's mind.

When someone does not self-identify as being disabled right away in the interaction, others sometimes report feeling a bit misled by the person's appearance, which promotes uneasiness and trust issues within the relationship. The individual may then hear, "What else is wrong with you?" or "You fooled me."

Scott, a friend of mine in college, found it hard to do the course readings outside of class because of his dyslexia. I asked him why he didn't take advantage of the support available. He confessed to me, "I don't want anyone to know, because I don't think I am strong enough to deal with the stigma that comes from having a disability."

Often, I will ask people with hidden disabilities who are too proud to reach out for access to support services to look at their lives critically. Which is worse: asking for help, receiving it, and getting on to bigger challenges in life? Or struggling and stumbling because friends and family to see them as weak or in a lesser light?

Before I was self-aware enough to recognize all the advantages of Disability Privilege given to me, my recognition of it existed because of other people noticing it for me. When I am with new people out in public, they will make comments like "Everybody is so nice to you" or "It's funny that homeless people don't ask you for money." I guess their assumption is that I should keep my money because I probably need it more than they do.

My experience with Disability Privilege has tainted my understanding about other people's experiences. I just assumed that people were always nice and friendly to each other. So, when they offered to help me out, this was not out of the ordinary.

Now I notice that the more progressive and diverse a city is—think Seattle, New York City, Portland, Austin, and San Francisco—the less Disability Privilege I receive. People don't go out of their way to interact with me and assist me with my daily tasks like they do in smaller cities. At first, I simply assumed they were less friendly. Then a friend of mine pointed out that they interacted with me in a more traditional way.

When people treat me like everyone else, I think something is wrong. I jokingly say that I am powered by status and validation. My Disability Privilege gives me both, and when it's gone, I miss it!

Amazing and inspirational work has been done by, and on behalf of, many famous celebrities. Many generations of people grew up watching Michael J. Fox on television and film as the good-looking, likeable, sympathetic person, to whom many could relate. Now we watch him push through his struggles with Parkinson's, all the while continuing to be a good servant for us. Even after he was diagnosed, he still pro-vided us with compelling stories and characters while leading, motivating, and inspir-ing us to overcome our challenges.

Christopher Reeve's portrayal of one of the most popular superhero characters of all time, Superman, is still relatable to able-bodied people today. Even toward the end of his life, suffering through the daily challenges of his existence, he seemed able to transcend these because he was someone with whom people could identify. As an actor, he showed us many different roles and faces over the years. People felt like they knew him, and that's why his presence can still be felt.

The hard work of both Fox and Reeve, combined with the impact of Disability Privilege, has allowed their charitable foundations to accomplish some amazing milestones on behalf of people in need.

At the time of this writing, the Michael J. Fox Foundation for Parkinson's Research was the largest nonprofit funder of Parkinson's disease research in the world. The Christopher and Dana Reeve Foundation, through June of 2016, has awarded 2,544 Quality of Life Grants totaling over $20.6 million. Since 1982 the foundation has invested $120 million into research.[1]

Truly life-changing amounts of good have been done with the money raised by these fine organizations. I can only imagine how amazingly good it must feel to serve as a personal vessel through which people can manifest their goodwill. What an honor and responsibility it is to use Disability Privilege to genuinely do good.

The perception of how someone has acquired their disability makes a huge difference as to how much Disability Privilege is given to them. For example, a person who lost a portion of their leg as a result of the 2013 Boston Marathon bombing will receive more Disability Privilege and help than a person who was driving drunk and lost a leg in an accident.

The victim of the bombing is seen by the general public as having a much more sympathetic acquisition story and will garner more goodwill and charitable resources, i.e., Disability Privilege, because of the perceived injustice that brought about how they became disabled. This is in contrast to someone who caused the injury themselves. The bombing victim will also have a greater chance to use their experience for good works and may be given the opportunity to serve as motivation for the general public.

As a result of my birth defect, I am able to make the most out of my own story. I have benefited from an incredible amount of goodwill received from strangers. Anyone could be faced with the consequences of having a child born without limbs. With that in mind, it is easier for able-bodied people to sympathize with my situation because they believe it could have been them.

---

1 https://www.christopherreeve.org/about-us/our-story

Because of the work I do, I find myself wishing for a better story to tell people, one that would provide me a larger platform to do more good work. I didn't cut my arm off on a hiking expedition out west. I wasn't injured working or fighting for truth, justice, and the American Way. Nobody did anything to take my legs away. I was just born without them. It is up to me to do as much good as I can with my own story. Maybe that's what everybody is trying to do with theirs.

Disability Privilege has an added benefit because of the times in which we live. Many times when people see I have no legs, they assume I lost my legs in active combat in a branch of the Armed Forces.

Once when shopping at a large retail store, I passed a man and a woman in their seventies. I smiled as they checked out my wheelchair. I gave them a quick smile and dip of my head to acknowledge their interest. They seemed to make the connection, and we were all on our way.

Throughout my shopping mission in the store, our paths crossed a few times. And, each time, we greeted each other with our eyes. We met up one final time at the checkout area. They were in line right behind me. I first felt a touch on my shoulder, and then I heard the woman's knowing voice. She must have mistaken me for someone else because she remarked, "Johansen?"

I turned around and met her eyes to confirm she was speaking to me. "No. Glowacki," I replied.

She looked down and said, "The war?"

I gave her the "I did it the easy way; I was just born without any" comeback.

What she said next surprised me: "This must be a really great time to be disabled."

What a truly insightful comment. For that older woman to recognize that there is no better time in the world to be disabled is a great comment and a powerful moment.

Twenty-five-plus years into the Americans with Disabilities Act (ADA), the physical infrastructure of our society has been modified to accommodate most physical disabilities. For the first time, people are going to work with the highest levels of assistive technologies. Attitudes and expectations are changing so quickly that people are no longer surprised to see me, a disabled person, out in public.

But then, she elaborated, "You probably get a lot of extra sympathy right now."

Well, she was right.

Positive social relevance and value have been placed on wounded warriors return-ing from the war. In her mind, the perception of society's reaction to the sacrifices veterans have made should create extra beneficial attention for anyone who could pass as being a veteran. As someone with a physical disability, it's easy to get swept up in Disability Privilege, but then it's up to me to respond appropriately.

Another reason why Disability Privilege is present and so pervasive in all groups in our society is because of the nature of disability, plus a general fear of one's own fragility. At any point, anyone has the unforeseen opportunity to join the minority group of "disabled."

The threat of joining our inclusive minority group generates immediate and additional empathy for our situation. People think: *That could be me someday.*

It's true—an able-bodied person can become disabled at any time. And within the disabled community, there is even a generalized acronym for able-bodied people. They are called *TABs*, or temporarily able-bodied. I find the term to be a bit crude, but the concept accurate. According to the Council for Disability Awareness, their research shows that "Just over 1 in 4 of today's 20 year olds will become disabled before they retire."[2]

POINT TO PONDER: What effect does visible celebrity disability have on the public perception of disabilities? Do you think Disability Privilege is given more to people born with disabilities or to people who acquired a disability?

The lengths taken by able-bodied people to avoid unintended membership in my minority group still surprises me. This next account still haunts me.

---

2 http://www.disabilitycanhappen.org/docs/disability_stats.pdf

After presenting my ideas at one college campus, a young veteran from the war in Iraq waited in line to speak to me. He shared a specific part of his military experience that really bothered him: While he was "in country," one of the initiation agreements passed on from veteran combat soldiers to the "new guys" was that if one's wounds were a "crippling" spinal cord injury, a head wound, or a genital wound, then his comrades in arms would take care of him by delivering a fatal headshot.

In essence, these young, strong heroes were told it is better for them to be dead than "crippled."

I am glad he shared his story with me, but it really made me upset, because of how short-sighted the perspectives of the other veterans were.

He explained to me, "I have a younger brother who was born with a disability that kept him from walking, but he uses a wheelchair and has a great life."

I could tell he was really troubled about that part of his fifteen-month tour, but he had never said anything because of the need to protect the "brothers in arms" agreement. I have heard similar stories too, often while listening in stunned disbelief.

A similar line of thinking appears to be at play when you look at the behavior demonstrated by parents when it comes to making a decision about prenatal screening. The underlying assumption in the discussion is possibly more disturbing. Based on the results of a test, parents are given the opportunity to consider the likelihood of having a child with a disability.

If the prenatal screening comes back as positive for some disorder or disability, the parents are then left to decide if they would be open to taking on the responsibility for a living, breathing, loving, developmentally disabled member of their family...or not. I consider myself and my family fortunate because my parents didn't find themselves having to making that kind of a decision, because no tests like that existed during the time of my mother's pregnancy.

Most able-bodied people are members of a "non-disabled, privileged" class. In the book *Privilege, Power, and Difference*, Allan G. Johnson actually creates the phrase

Non-Disabled Privilege to refer to the privilege of not being burdened with the stigma and subordinated status that goes along with being identified as disabled.

Within the previous explanation of the phrase is the assumption that member-ship in the group or class of people with a disability immediately lowers a person's societal status and their access to advantages and benefits of the culture.

When interacting with able-bodied people, I feel the presence of an understated thankfulness from them because of an internalized appreciation they have for what they believe I must be going through. Through the words they use when speaking to me and how they act when they are around me, it feels as if their perception is that I am shouldering a burden for them because they do not have to experience what I am experiencing. For example, during conversations with me, people like to highlight and reflect on all the things they think I can't do. Yes, life is still hard. I will not deny the existence of additional, daily challenges arising from my unique circum-stances. But I would rather have someone assume my life is meaningful and that I can do anything, than assume it is barely worth living and they have to take care of me because it is the right thing to do.

CHAPTER 3
Entitlement

Just like my friends at college in the 1990s who took advantage of Disability Privilege and over-accommodation, I also found myself developing a sense of entitlement.

In high school, my cousin Terry and I were shooting at cans with BB guns when I jokingly pumped up my gun while he was resetting the cans, making him feel like I was going to take aim at him. He quickly responded to my actions by saying, "If you shoot at me, don't think that I'm not going to shoot you back just because you don't have any legs."

I scoffed. "What do you mean?"

He straightened up and looked at me. "You're entitled."

He explained what he meant: I had adopted entitlement when it came to not being held responsible for doing something wrong. Often, people are slow to blame a person with a disability for anything they do incorrectly. I shrugged him off and forgot his comments.

A few years later in college, when friends and I were visiting a bar to watch the football game, I started criticizing a visiting fan of the opposing team. The situation escalated, and I turned around toward my friends to step up for me and handle any part of the physical altercation I was anticipating. They backed me up and we all avoided a very potentially harmful and charged situation. But afterward, my friend Jason led our group of people outside to have a talk.

He confronted me in front of everyone, saying, "Just because we are with you doesn't mean we are always going to be **with** you."

He told me not to run my mouth because one of these times I'd deserve to feel the real consequences of my actions. I knew he was my friend because he held me to the same standard as all his other friends. I respected him for not being afraid to look insensitive for making me accountable.

Many times, my disability has served me as a shield from the consequences of my actions. Very few people not hold me to the same standard of behavior to which they hold able-bodied people. That might sound like an advantage in many situations, but I have come to learn it often isn't, especially because of the friends it has cost me.

Looking back, I now know that I have lost people in my life because it was easier for them to just stop being present than to confront me about my actions. Without realizing it, I was taking advantage of my privilege and hiding behind my wheelchair. I was using privilege to get me out of negatively charged situations that I had started.

This issue is something that I still struggle with and am constantly working on. I try never to put someone else in a situation where they will have to fight a battle on my behalf. In all aspects of life, I never ask someone to do something for me that I would not do for myself if at all possible. Luckily, I have wonderful partners and a strong group of friends who show me every day what a good friend looks like, and they give me the chance to be one. It wasn't until many years later, and after several experiences, that I learned this lesson: Being disabled brings with it a sense of entitlement due to Disability Privilege.

I enjoy being able to drive into any parking lot and know that there is almost a 100 percent chance I will be able to have a special place in the front reserved for me. It is not my best characteristic, but I feel entitled to those spots.

Even when other vehicles with appropriate credentials take them, I feel short-changed that I can't use the space there for me. Immediately, I start wondering just how disabled these people are. Are they persons who use wheelchairs and need the extra footage in the space or are they just fakers who stole someone else's placard?

Handicapped parking is an example of a priority service given to people with disabilities. When I notice a car (like police cruisers, delivery vehicles, or service vehicles) is parked illegally without the credential, it means to me that someone has determined that the vehicle's context trumps my needs.

Businesses recognize the value able-bodied people place in priority parking. I have seen a reduction in the number of handicapped parking places and the re-designation of our spaces for "elite status" members of hotel chains or for hybrid or electric car owners. It is fine to want to accommodate and recognize people for their status, but violating the spirit of accessibility to honor and reward others doesn't seem correct to me.

Handicapped parking is the most visible, public accommodation made for people with disabilities. Generally, able-bodied people understand and buy into the importance of the spaces but can justify anything during inclement weather. I always notice how everyone seems to be disabled when it rains.

When traveling between two different presentations, I was in the middle of Ohio and needed a gas station to use the bathroom. I parked at a pump. As I pushed the driver's side rear sliding door button on my dash, the door opened. I turned around in my seat, grabbed and removed my wheelchair from the empty space where the rear passenger seating would be, and transferred myself onto my wheelchair to fill the tank.

The ADA allows people who have disabilities to request access assistance from the gas station attendant. In many cases, there are buttons on the pumps, or stickers with the local phone number of the exact station to call to alert them to your need of help. The attendant is required by law to come out and pump gas at no additional cost to the individual with the disability. The law, however, is interpreted very differently by each station—and from what I understand, in talking to other people with disabilities, very differently from employee to employee at the stations.

I have never taken advantage of that accommodation because, even on the coldest day or in the rainiest weather, my disability causes no more trouble to me than anyone else when it comes to pumping my own gas. I can understand why that law exists for people who might not be able to exit their vehicle because of space require- ments for their ramps or related equipment.

After I finished filling my tank, I headed toward the gas station door. In the back, doors with the universal male and female bathroom signs were accompanied with *Employees Only* signs. I inquired with the attendant about the location of their bath- rooms, and she told me they were outside.

I made my way out and was unpleasantly surprised, and also taken aback. The management had decided to employ two porta-toilets alongside the building instead of offering traditional restrooms. The only saving grace was that the larger porta-toilet was designed for a wheelchair user, and it had a ramp.

As I was about ten feet away, a girl rushed ahead of me, grabbed the door of the larger toilet to open it for herself. I immediately spoke up and made mention to her that there were two options, but only one I could use because of my disability. She quickly exclaimed, "I have claustrophobia!"

She entered and slammed the door.

I have to admit, I was mad. But I didn't scream at her, I didn't bang on the door, and I didn't use my car to push over the porta-toilet. Although many of those things crossed my mind.) I just waited my turn.

She finished and opened the door, averting her eyes from mine as she walked by me to get into her Toyota Prius with a handicapped parking permit in the window.

I should have let it go, but this interaction caused me to think about how I felt and why I felt like I did. I immediately did the math of who needed it more based on what I determined to be "real" need. I can admit that if she really did have claustrophobia, using the larger one would be a legitimate need because of her disability.

It wasn't until after these experiences that I recognized my entitlement, brought about by Disability Privilege. But just as some offered me Disability Privilege, others judged me.

CHAPTER 4

Assumptions

have found that people in general often mean the best, but they can be wholly misinformed about disabilities or anything outside the norm.

What still surprises me is the effect that two people in wheelchairs have on the public. Sometimes it's people who just want to walk by and chime in, but it makes me crazy when they say, "Hey, are you guys racing?" or "One of you is going to get a speeding ticket!"

Other comments range from, "It is great to see you guys out together" or "Are you guys related?"

My favorite comment is when someone sees me next to another male in a wheelchair and asks, "What's wrong with your brother?" The *only* commonality we have is the fact that we use wheelchairs.

That perception does come in handy, though, when I'm out with another person who uses a wheelchair and I need to find him. I can go up to anyone and ask, "Have you seen my brother?" Ninety-nine percent of the time, they direct me right to the place where he was last spotted.

On one of my recent tours, I parked my rental car—a brand new, dark blue Honda Civic—in one of the handicapped parking spots at Wal-Mart. Membership does have its privileges! I knew getting in and out of this particular vehicle was going to be a little more challenging than just grabbing my wheelchair out of the side door of my minivan.

When traveling by myself, I often choose the most cost-effective option of a smaller rental car. I opt for cost savings over convenience, but it does require me to take the large wheels off my chair and place them in the back seat of the car. Then, I lift the large seat structure part of the frame over my body and place it in the passenger seat next to me. It is more cumbersome than anything and it usually takes upwards of thirty seconds to a minute to load and unload my chair from the car.

That day, the amount of time required to reassemble my chair was just enough to draw a crowd of people entering and exiting the store. The crowd captured the atten-tion of the store's greeter.

The greeter came to find out what was happening, but by the time he exited the store and started to make his way toward me, I was already on my chair moving with the crowd toward the front doors.

I met him just outside the door, and we had a conversation.

He paid me a compliment, saying, "Wow, it is amazing that you can do that yourself!"

With a bit of harmless sarcasm, I responded by saying, "Thank you, and you walk very well."

I'd hoped that he would have gotten the compliment I intended, relating it to how we both are good at what we do all the time.

But then he continued, "Who brought you here?"

I replied politely, "I did. There's no one with me and I exited on the driver's side of the vehicle."

He exclaimed, "Wow. It's amazing you can drive a car—because you're in a wheelchair."

I said, "No, it's not that amazing. I do it all the time."

He reiterated, "It is a miracle that you can do it by yourself."

He congratulated me on my accomplishments, and we both went our separate ways.

I don't have a problem with the entire conversation. I appreciate questions and comments, I really do. After all, people are intrigued by things and people that are different. Plus, since there are few people like me in the world, in some unique way, I represent the handicapped community to them. I want and need people to have that positive experience, to have the conversation and ask the questions. This prevents them from making up their own answers and misinforming other people.

The problem I have with the conversation, though, is when he said, "It's amazing you can drive a car—because you're in a wheelchair."

I view it as an ignorant or uninformed statement. Not ignorant in an offensive, malicious way, but understandably ignorant in terms of a lack of insight into another person's life experience and a simple misunderstanding of someone's potential.

But I have to look at it in a different way. His statement "It's amazing you can drive a car" could almost come off as a compliment. In fact, in his mind, I'm sure it was.

The greeter made mention of an accomplishment that seemed extraordinary to him. Perhaps in his mind, it is the same as congratulating someone for climbing a tall mountain, and accomplishing it all while dealing with a tremendous amount of effort, when in fact, driving a car for me is far easier than pushing a wheelchair.

The initial accomplishment could be noteworthy, but my problem is with the perception of how valid the accomplishment is in context. Many times, the perception of this "accomplishment" is based on the person paying the compliments. When the person pays a compliment to the other person, many times it reflects a lower expectation because of their limited experiences.

Compare the first statement about driving to a parallel statement that many people might find also to be ignorant. "Wow. It's amazing you can drive a car—because you're in a wheelchair" is comparable to "Wow. It's amazing you're in college because you're a woman."

Congratulating a woman on attending college is silly because we know being a woman is not a disadvantage to intelligence or academics. Although it wasn't always the belief, today society knows that both men and women are equally competent to do well in institutions of higher learning.

Complimenting a woman for going to college today might appear that the person delivering the compliment has a lower expectation of them. That's the same argu-ment when complimenting the person with the disability.

Is it correct to make mention of how someone else accommodates their situation if we find it to be ingenious or interesting? Of course. But, the words a person uses make all the difference when we are trying to establish the context and understanding of another person's experience.

If you want to know if I can drive or how that actually works, just ask, but phrase the question in a way that doesn't suppose inability or a judgement made because of a stereotype. You could say, "I assume you can drive, but how does that work?"

And if you want to know, I hold the steering wheel with my right hand at about the two o' clock position. It allows me to direct the car with small movements up and down. I palm the wheel to go around corners. My left hand is always resting on my hand controls—I refer to them as glorified pedal extensions, pieces of steel rod that extend to the floor and clamp on to the pedals with wing nuts. There is a right-angle handgrip on the rod for the brake pedal, and next to it, the rod that controls the gas. The top of that gas rod has a round button I apply pressure to with my thumb to ac-celerate. Everything works perfectly as long as I don't push the gas and the brake at the same time, or there could be problems!

POINT TO PONDER: Have you ever had someone place a stereotype on you that assumed you were limited in what you could do? How did it make you feel? If you had a chance to educate them about that stereotype, what would you say?

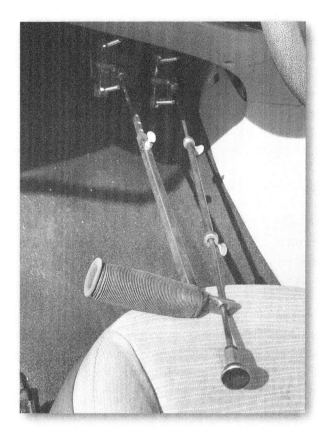

Too often, society places stereotypes others because people don't know enough about others' situations. This is true for me, of course, and it's true for many other people as well.

I attended a conference recently and listened to a session from an African American woman named Evonne. She said that she constantly witnessed small micro-aggressions in people's language and behavior toward her. To illustrate her point, she shared a few examples to people in the audience. People often tell her that she doesn't act like a normal black person, they try to touch her hair, or her personal favorite is when people tell her, "You're really pretty for a person with dark skin."

As people began to understand her predicament, everyone wanted to know how she kept such a positive manner when she was with people, even though it seemed as if she was under constant attack.

Evonne understood She wasn't living in a majority culture made for her. She was just a tourist, and people who engaged in those behaviors weren't trying to attack her; they just weren't seeing the world from her perspective. Because they were different from her, they didn't know what she went through because they had no idea how to relate to her life. Their reactions and perceptions of her culture hurt her feelings sometimes, but she tries to measure people's intentions instead of the impact their ignorance has on her experience.

The person committing the micro-aggression is most likely unaware of the inappropriateness of their interaction; very rarely are these interactions purposefully designed to be hurtful. However, the discrimination created by the micro-aggression is still present and real. Evonne blames the negative impact of the micro-aggression on the larger problems of cultural institutionalized racism, not the person who com-mits the act.

She said that perspective helps her maintain positive relationships with people outside of her culture. When Evonne has a chance to explain to her colleagues and friends how what they said to her could be considered less than helpful, those people say thank you for broadening their understanding of what other people have to go through based on who they are.

Although my experiences as a person with a disability are completely different than hers as a black woman, I feel the same way she does concerning micro-aggressions. In my mind, the context rhymes.

Have you ever been somewhere where English is not a spoken language? Each time during the day, as the language barrier causes inconveniences, it feels frustrating. When individuals feel out of place in their own homeland, that less-than-ideal experience can be caused by the negative effects of privilege.

I feel like a tourist in my own land, although the ADA was supposed to have fixed that. There are laws that have removed physical barriers I could consider micro-aggressions like curbs and steps, but those laws have only been around for twenty-five years. The infrastructure and society of the US have been around for over 200. Today, I still see myself that way because I have recognized I don't have legs, and things aren't always designed for me.

My life before the ADA was difficult. But I didn't know it was hard, because the way I did things was normal around my supportive family. I was ignorant to my situation and how it could have been because of the absence of my legs.

I didn't really know how having legs would make things much more convenient. Yet, during the day I could see my friends play soccer or carry each other around on their shoulders, but without even the chance of me having real functional legs, I never felt it as that much of a daily injustice. I was focused on how to get what I wanted with what I had.

I've had a ton of experiences, which, for the most part, have been near what they actually should be, and probably had many more total experiences than average people. I find solace in that, knowing that I have been to more places, seen more things, and met more people than most others. I think that Disability Privilege has provided me the opportunity to get access to more experiences too. In order for me to have those experiences, I have to operate in a world that is not meant for me.

Every day I am met with challenges that make it harder for me to do something and put me in a place where I have to admit and demonstrate to people I am physically in a worse situation than they might be. But if I stayed in my perfect completely accessible house, had my groceries delivered, and my bills paid by the government, I might not feel as disabled because I wasn't running into broken elevators or dealing with ignorant people who try to give me money or hit on my girlfriend because they assume she would never be with me. Also, I'd never have seen Broadway musicals, been ATVing in the Painted Desert, or had great sex in really inaccessible public places - which makes it even more fun.

I felt less like a tourist when I was young because I belonged in my family, in my home, in my schools, and with my friends, and everyone tried to include me all the time. I was included so I wasn't an "other." I just had to do things in a different way.

These days, I travel mostly by myself. There isn't a set of people who are trying to include me. I have to do all that work myself. When I see a curb, I have to deal with it. No one is there before me cutting the curb or telling me where to go to avoid it. People see me accommodating myself and say things like, "We didn't think any of you guys would be here" or "We never realized it wouldn't work for wheelchair people."

Every day, I am aware of things I can't use or that won't work for me, and people say ignorant things to me. I don't know if they are all micro-aggressions, but I can see how someone might call it that.

Each situation depends on my interpretation of the challenge in the moment. If I am at your house and your backyard gate isn't wide enough for my wheelchair, I'm not going to get angry at you. However, if I'm at IKEA and their cart fence has a large thirty-six-inch wide gate in it. Next to the gate, there's a button that says *Push for service if in a wheelchair* and I push it for five minutes and nothing happens. When I go into the customer service desk and inquire about it, and they say, "Yeah that doesn't work because it broke, and we didn't fix it because it is easier for us to have handicapped people come and ask for help out to your car," I look at that more as a negative attack. I believe I should be able to have free and easy access in and out of a big box retailer just like an able-bodied person.

When an incident like that frustrates me, it's because it makes me look more disabled to someone else because I need more help than I should. Yet, I try to put that away and look at it like "I need to do my job and find the person who is in charge of facilities at IKEA and sell them a speech about intention and accessibility." Because of how and when I was raised, it invigorates me more than it shuts me down.

The ADA has been wonderful in allowing me freedom to live a life as close to being able-bodied as possible. However, the tiny interruptions, however—mostly from people who underestimate what I'm capable of doing—do add up.

Still, I want to be the black woman who sees the injustice, identifies it, and tries not to let it get her down or let it keep her from getting what she wants. For me, this the best possible life—full of treasures, experiences, and love. If I stay at home and never interact with the world because my feelings get hurt or things are inconvenient for me, that will make me far more disabled than not having legs.

Life is hard for me, but life is hard for plenty of able-bodied people as well. We all have a purpose, a skill, and even our own version of a disability. I see not having legs as a minor issue. How people respond to me as "less than" is the bigger disability to me. Their thinking that way, I believe, is a disability for them. It's experiences like these that make me feel like a tourist in my own country.

CHAPTER 5

The Judgment Game

A friend of mine once told me, "The story you make up about me, tells me more about you than it does me."

When I am making my way through a restaurant or visiting a store, people stop talking to each other or look up from what they are doing and pay attention to me. I guess my presence within their proximity is a better story or more interesting than what they are doing. Maybe they're surprised I'm out in the world on my own—that I'm *capable*. Hopefully, I can surprise some people with how I live my life day to day. As a guy who built a public speak-ing career through my disability, I guess that attention is probably good for business.

I was in a hotel lobby in Spokane when a woman stepped in front of me, stopping me in my tracks, and said, "You look like my cousin, 'cause he was just in a car accident and has to use a wheelchair. But don't worry—he's going to get better."

When the woman made her comment, she had already made a few assumptions about me. She made them without having any actual information besides what she could see. She related to me through an experience she had with someone close to her, and my mere existence caused her to connect both of us. I have to believe she possibly thought she was paying me a compliment or at least relating to me on some level.

Unfortunately, her comment about her cousin getting better stung me. I under-stand that she could have been coming to grips with her family member's newfound disability. But to me, her comment implied that walking is better than having to use a wheelchair to get around. It may have been better for him because of his primary experience of walking up to that point versus having to use a wheelchair only for his recovery.

It is also a wildly ignorant thing for her to say because it reflects no actual knowledge about the quality of my life. Her statement that her cousin is going to "get better" and get out of the wheelchair implies that her cousin's life will soon be better than mine. What she failed to realize is that this is my life—there is no "getting better" for me. And, my life is just fine.

Her concept of "better" and my concept of "better" are in no way related or connected, not to mention that her cousin's accident and my disability are in no way connected. I can only assume that she used the standard able-bodied metric of "the ability to walk is a major part of a good quality of life."

By now you know I think otherwise.

Her comment also reminded me that I was different. I understand that she was probably trying to bridge a gap and relate to me, but it only reinforced my "other" status in my mind.

I tried not to let it bother me, but I felt as though I needed to prove to her that my life was meaningful and pleasurable to justify me wanting to live it. But why should I try to prove and justify myself to a stranger?

POINT TO PONDER: Have you ever felt like you had to justify part of your life to someone, just to be accepted?

I always had at least a little reverence for what I was taught in Sunday school. I thought the selected versions of the stories shared from the Bible were, for the most part, fair. I was always impressed with how just and accepting God was portrayed to be, and how we all fit into God's plan. We were all told that we were made in God's image. I came to believe it and lived my life with that understanding. None of us are perfect, but we are all children of God.

That is why I'm surprised when I'm out in public and some self-professed Christian approaches me and inquires about the nature of my disability. When I tell them, I was born without legs, they always say something along the lines of "You know, I'm a Christian, and I just wanted to tell you I'm really sorry for what happened to you."

I always ask them, "Why?"

They usually say something like "I am sorry God made you like that."

With great restraint, I resist the temptation to snap back, "And I am sorry God made you like *that!*"

No matter how many times I hear it, I'm always stunned by what they say. It goes against everything I was ever taught about why God works in the ways that He does. Isn't God's love unconditional?

When people approach me with this line of reasoning, I say, "I didn't think God made mistakes."

Most of the time they all reply with "That isn't what I meant by that…"

And then they'll end with "I'll pray for you."

I always thank them, because in saying, "I'll pray for you," they must perceive it to be their job. They are also probably trying to offer me some kind of comfort to make me feel better. I don't need them to try to make me feel better. Honestly, I feel just fine. Thank you.

Their use of words to make me feel "better" implies that my current situation is worse than theirs. You know what? It might be to them. But I was born without legs, and I am working as hard as I can with my experience to find my peace of mind, just like they are.

I usually end up having a conversation with them about how I believe that everyone is born with unique abilities and opportunities based on their situation. Most of the time, however, all they want to do is talk about all of the things they are sure I can't do. With empathy, they try to commiserate with me because of my situation as they perceive it.

It is almost as if they missed attending a pity party I surely must have held for the absence of my legs, and now they want to make up for it. But I never threw that party. And there was never any pity. I do not need or want to pretend to feel something I don't just to help them relate to a false situation they created in their mind.

It's not my job to make them feel okay with the fact that I do not have legs. However, I don't want them to leave our interaction with the misinformation of my life being sad and so much worse than theirs. But it isn't my job to convince someone else that my life is all right either.

In my mind, if there is a God, he did not make a mistake when he made me. I'm doing fine; I have been at this for quite a while now, and I'm pretty good at it.

I draw parallels to the situation of a friend of mine named Scott. Tragically, he lost his first wife and baby girl in a car accident. Now, years later, he has remarried.

When he meets people for the first time, he does everything he can to avoid disclosing the very private and still painful experience of the death of his first wife and child. But when it comes up, he also doesn't want to appear standoffish or aloof. He simply shares his story as quickly and succinctly as possible and tries to move on from the conversation.

After he shares the short version of the story, people aren't wrong for trying to apologize for asking the question and trying to offer what I am sure they think are supportive com-ments like "You are so amazing for going through a tragedy like that" or "I could never get over losing my spouse and first child."

He typically thanks them for their concern, and then he tries to change the sub-ject. But people often don't want to let it go. They want to fully engage with him about how much of a loss he must have felt. They try to sympathize, too, by sharing their own personal, tragic stories with him.

Continuing the conversation forces him to do even more work to reassure them that he is all right now, even if he isn't. It causes him to experience a sliver of the pain again. He tries to downplay and minimize the personal impact he feels. Scott said to try to get out of the situation, he puts on that he has healed from the loss, even if it hurts him to have to minimize its impact.

As I talked to him about this at great length, he explained to me how he doesn't want it to be his job to constantly make people feel better about a personal tragedy he suffered over twenty years ago. Similarly, I wish I didn't have the burden of attempting to convince everyone that I am doing fine and trying to overcome my disability every day. We both try not to allow our situations to impact other people. We don't want to be viewed as "victims" by others. We just want to blend in—it's easier and much more painless. No, I don't want a pity party. But sometimes, I find that other people really want to host one for me.

POINT TO PONDER: Have you ever had to minimize the impact of a personal tragedy, just so you did not have to explain it again and relive the pain?

I am still surprised how many people make judgements about my ex-wife. I was married to a wonderful woman named Shannon for four years. Our relationship ended because our lives were going in different directions, and we both agreed to split up and pursue our own interests. But when she comes up in conversation, people often assumed that she used a wheelchair to get around, too. I guess when they think of a couple being in love and getting married, with one person using a wheelchair, they figure both people must be "confined" to them. When I explain that she did not need or use one, many times people actually say, "Well, good for you," as if I'm "lucky" to have suckered someone who's not a wheelchair user into marrying me.

Those moments still show me that people's misconceptions and assumptions lead to their judging me inaccurately. I started to wonder how many times I had made the same mistake when interacting with other people. How did my assumptions about them change my words and actions based on the limited amount of information I had?

It bothered me so much, I decided to create an exercise through which I would be able to help people explore their own "judgmental value system." I wanted to see how the stories people make up about strangers might affect the ways they interact with people who are different from them, especially if the difference could be perceived externally. I decided to conduct these discussions primarily with my college audiences in my role as a public speaker. I called it the "Judgment Game."

I have found that most people like talking about dating and the impact it has on their life. So, I began the discussion by asking each person to share with the group an example of a characteristic that someone could exhibit that would be an immediate "red flag" that would stop you from dating them—a deal breaker.

I explained that, to me, "smoking cigarettes" is not an acceptable answer because currently most college students in the United States look at it as unhealthy and unacceptable. Basically, it's not a good indicator of someone's value system; people view it as more of an unattractive habit. The best examples are of an intrinsic human charac-teristic or consequence versus a personal behavior or behavioral choice.

One student claimed that all of their partners *have* to love dogs or the outdoors. If the person they were interested in didn't share in those loves, it would serve as a disqualifier to them.

Other students said things like their potential partners would have to have a college degree or have a great job. I soon began to notice that the more comfortable the group felt with each other, the more personal the demands became. By having people share their disqualifiers, you can also really learn about a person's history and culture.

I decided to share one last good example with this group before they started. I told them about discussing this exercise with a friend of mine who shared one of his deal breakers: He would never be able to date someone who was HIV positive. This surprised me because with current forms of treatment and survival success rates of those living with HIV and AIDS, I didn't think it was that big of a deal anymore. I asked him why and he said, "The fact that he has the diagnosis proves that he makes poor decisions, and I don't want to have to worry about contracting it myself."

His comment showed me another dimension of stereotypes that still exist surrounding HIV. However, it gave me the perfect transition into the next part of the exercise.

After everyone explained most of their disqualifiers and their reasons behind them, I asked them to come up with the one situation where their potential partner could exhibit that characteristic, but it would not serve as a disqualifier.

For example, a person who is allergic to cats might still be willing to cohabitate with a cat owner and take medicine and negotiate cat-free zones in their residence, while still experiencing hardship to be with their partner.

Students who had refused to even consider people who didn't meet their standard were now considering how they might be devaluing other potential mates. They were now forced to think about how their life could exist with their "perfect" companion and their "imperfect" stereotype.

As the discussion continued, some students in the group talked about how they had actually been with people who exhibited some of those disqualifying characteristics. Then, they also shared what they did to minimize their differences, so they could be together. The group started to see that many of the characteristics a person might think could be disqualifying could actually be overcome.

At the end of the activity, I shared with students the rest of the story about my friend who claimed he wouldn't date someone with HIV.

I explained how when I asked my friend to come up with a situation where he would be willing to date someone who was living with the HIV diagnosis, he said that the person would have had to acquire it through a blood transfusion during childhood. I was still bothered by his answer, but we continued the conversation.

A few weeks later, he approached me at a gallery opening. He had done some more research about people living with HIV and AIDS, and he wanted to let me know he was wrong for making decisions about things he didn't fully understand. He thanked me for broadening his perspectives and helping to educate him.

As the students in the activity spoke about my friend's realization, they all understood how easy it was for them to be scared off by their own incorrect assumptions without having any real information or reasons to see past a perceived disqualifying characteristic.

Finally, I shared with the students that it is okay for everyone to have standards and expectations for the people they let into their lives. It's all right to keep people at arm's length based on their histories of violence, theft, or other kinds of abuse. It's okay to be selective.

I explained that I was just trying to challenge them into paying a little more attention to the next time they quickly disqualify someone from their life based on an outward characteristic, a stereotype, or an uninformed story they create and believe to be true without any context or understanding of who that person is—or more importantly, who that person could be.

I don't like to be judged on the quality of my life, and I wouldn't want to do that to others. That's why it surprised me when I judged a friend of mine poorly who voluntarily chose to get a five-by-ten bright blue handicapped parking sign tattooed on his chest. I asked him why he chose that image, and he told me that it was a self-portrait. Aghast, I told him, "You might use a wheelchair, but that's just an outward character-istic. It isn't who you are!"

Unmoved by my comment, he simply said, "I'm handicapped."

I didn't realize later that when I told him that being handicapped was not who he was, I was actually telling him to deny and reject his own identity as he perceived it. It's important to step back and realize that people's self-perceptions are different. What I may find true about myself is not necessarily true for others. I was upset with my friend's new tattoo because I was trying to protect the person I thought I needed to be. I want to not be seen as handicapped and to be accepted by the larger society of which I am a part. I assumed that's what he wanted too—when that wasn't the case.

POINT TO PONDER: Have you ever judged someone as less than or unworthy because of a characteristic they displayed? Did you have an additional experience with that person which clarified their behavior in your mind or were your judgements proven to be incorrect? How did you handle that situation?

CHAPTER 6
Diversity Quicksand

A s I developed an understanding of why people judged me and my abilities based on their first visual perception of me, I also learned another thing: I judge others, too. I have spent my whole life preaching about how terrible it is for people to stereotype me just because I have a wheelchair. But I've been just as guilty of judging other people based on my perception of stereotypes as well.

I was presenting one of my motivational lectures on the campus of Eastern Kentucky University for their freshman orientation. About halfway through the program, I shared a story I frequently experience at the shopping mall around the Christmas season.

I explained how people who don't even know me approach me and hand me cash. It happens enough now that I can see it coming from a mile away. Usually the person sizes me up, they get a concerned look on their face, and they approach me while going for their wallet. Of course, I am ready for them by the time they start to speak. I start with "That is so very nice of you, but really, I am totally fine."

Insistent, they often reply, "No, this is for you."

I reply, "Really, I'm good—I'm not selling pencils or ringing a bell. Please keep your money."

If they persist, I take the money. I have come to learn that at that point, their giving me money is probably not even about me—it's about something they feel they need to do.

I actually made $81 this last holiday season, down from $123 the year before. I guess we're still in the recession.

After sharing the story with the audience, I knew I was making an impact. They hung on my every word. I was on a roll, quite literally, and I was looking forward to the question and answer portion of my event to really get to the meatier insights with the audience.

A couple of questions into the session, an African American woman approached the microphone and said she had more of a comment than a question. This was not unusual because, many times, people will preface their statements before they pay me a compliment. I was ready and willing to accept. Then, she surprised me by telling me that she had come to a new truth in her life. She stated, "I would rather be you than me."

I was a bit taken aback by what she said, and so I asked, "What do you mean?"

She said, "You are a white male without legs, using a wheelchair. And, from what you said, when you go to the mall, people come up and give you money, right?"

I said, "Yes, that is correct."

She continued, "I would rather be you than me, because as a black female, when I go to the mall, people think I'm going to steal."

I immediately tried to do what I thought was right—minimizing the impact of what she said and addressing her situation by saying, "That can't possibly be true."

In that moment, I realized just how wrong I was. I changed my tactic and said, "Thank you for sharing your experience and point of view. It is just as valid as mine. I want to understand your perspective and you have helped me do so. Obviously, I too need to spend more time finding out what the advantages and disadvantages are for any person who is a member of any minority group."

"However," I went on, "let me say this: We are as alike as we are different. Yet you say you would pick my life. Perhaps confronted with another set of life's travails, you might not. And the same goes for me. I might pick portions of your life to live and not others. I am sorry that untrue stereotypes and prejudices about African Americans force you into having to live that situation every day. It was my mistake when I denied your experience."

I was guilty of developing my own assumptions, generalizations, and stereotypes about other people's experiences and interactions with minority groups. I was doing exactly what I tell other people not to do—I was drawing conclusions about other people's quality of life and experiences based on my own perception of what their life must be like.

I developed those ideas about others from my own experience of multiple iden-tities, thus giving me a false understanding of her perspective. I am a white male, straight, with a disability. From what I could quickly glean from her appearance, she was a black, female, able-bodied, and enrolled in college.

What I needed to remember in the beginning of my interaction with her was that we are all members of multiple groups. As we all explore our own intersectionality, most of us belong to many dominant and subdominant groups.

The sharing of her experience with me should have been the perfect opportunity for me to empathize with her, exercise better listening skills, and take the time to ask more questions about what she was trying to tell me. I learned that equal access to experiences and places may look different depending on which minority and class you belong to.

My own access to and comfort with my situation clouded my judgment, how-ever. I made false determinations about her experiences because of the privileges I had come to take for granted, which were derived from the context of my own disability. As a white male, I have never been suspected or stereotyped of being a shoplifter. Her experience is something that, because of my circumstances, I cannot understand.

POINT TO PONDER: Have you ever misjudged someone else's experiences be-cause you made a determination about them based on a stereotype?

In every one of my audiences, there are people with great energy and agree-able smiles. I look for them and use them as emotional anchors. It is great to receive positive reinforcement from audience members. When I am not getting it, I worry that I'm not doing a good job.

Recently, I was speaking to students at a university in Georgia. As I approached the stage, I noticed there were fewer than fifty people in the audience. But that didn't stop me from receiving great feedback and energy from the people who were there. I noticed that on the right side of the audience, there sat a gentleman with an athletic build and a great smile. He seemed to really be enjoying himself because he nodded and affirmed every point I made. Sitting on the left side of the audience, though, was another man who was obviously not enjoying anything I said. I could tell because he never made eye contact with me or even chose to raise his head. The entire time, he didn't acknowledge anything that I said or did on stage. And, honestly, I was more than a little put off by it.

At the end of the presentation, the event coordinator approached me and asked me how I thought it went. I told her I thought that most of the people seemed to be with me, but I identified the two audience members I noticed.

"I wished the gentleman on the right would have toned it down a bit because his nodding in agreement with everything I said was just a bit distracting. And I was upset that I couldn't seem to connect with the guy on the left, because he would never make eye contact with me."

She said, "Well, that would be hard for both of them to do because Charles (on the right) has autism and Michael (on the left) is legally blind."

I couldn't have been more embarrassed. As a speaker myself, who teaches how to interact with people with disabilities, I totally got busted for making completely incorrect judgements.

I call this moment "Diversity Quicksand". It occurs when people, even with the best of intentions, fall into hard conversations or potentially hurtful situations after they make an inappropriate comment and/or misunderstand another person's situation. Almost everything they could or would say probably isn't going to make it any better. It's best not to struggle too much; the effort might just sink the entire interaction.

A more formal definition of "Diversity Quicksand" could be: when something is said or done during a conversation and it appears to lack sensitivity to someone or a minority group. It makes a larger negative impression when the person tries to fight, squirm, or read-just their wording to make it better. The situation only becomes worse because of questioned intentions, false motivation, and a perceived lack of sensitivity. Most people in our society will find themselves in that situation from time to time.

After speaking to a friend of mine named Sarah about the perils of Diversity Quicksand, she confessed to me, "Many times I choose not to speak to people who are different than me, because I don't want to even risk saying something that could hurt their feelings."

What she didn't realize was that *not* engaging with people who are different than herself could possibly do more damage to our society than her taking that risk. I said to her, "We need greater dialog and more groups of people understanding each other now more than ever."

I wish we could all agree on a "best assumption rule" for our interactions with other people. By this I mean that when we are speaking to another person, I hope that both parties could assume that neither one is trying to hurt the other person's feelings with their choice of words. I have met very few, if any, people who are trying to be cordial or want to be my friend that have intentionally tried to hurt my feelings by saying the wrong thing.

When people use an insensitive word to describe my disability—or me—I try to understand the context and their intent before I respond. I recognize that they are entering into a potentially high-risk conversation with me, but I'd rather have people talk to me and include me rather than ignore me to avoid possibly hurting my feelings.

If they do say something that triggers me, I respond, "I'm sure you didn't mean anything by what you just said, but because of my circumstance, when you said that, it made me feel like..."

Then I ask them, "Are there words or subject matters that you would share with me that, from your experience, could make you react in the same sort of way?"

I find that if I alert them when it happens, it prevents me from harboring ill will or making negative judgments about them without understanding the full context of their experience. Having that honest conversation strengthens the relationship, builds trust, and is a good lead into larger ideas about what is important to other people.

Everyone isn't my friend yet, and I recognize that strangers don't know how to refer to me and my experiences. It isn't fair for me to judge someone based on their words if they don't have the same definition of the words that I do. However, many times people will make moral judgments about a person, possibly labeling them in a pejorative way because they don't know the "right" word to use.

Most who engage in the study of diversity act as though their expertise comes with an additional moral high ground concerning the judgment of others. It doesn't. At the same time, many diversity professionals tell everyone they have to understand and accept something they never can understand, simply because of who they are. This leaves no comfortable space for anyone to even start having that conversation.

To protect themselves, members of the majority culture avoid conversations with diverse people because they perceive an implied threat of being called "racist" or "in-sensitive." But being afraid to openly talk with other people regarding these issues only hinders how we connect to each other across our differences. I am still not the best at this either. But I keep working to be understanding and help bring people to the hard conversations from where they are, trying to be a good friend to them along the way.

PART 3

Acceptance

CHAPTER 1

Dating

I have learned a few things about life. We might have different backgrounds or come from different cultures. I might not have legs, and I might have different colored skin than you. But I have learned that we are all people, and most of us want to be loved and accepted.

It saddens me to say that not everybody sees or values others in this way.

This is especially true in dating.

The presence of a disability could be a characteristic in some people's minds that would prevent them from seeing a person as a potential partner. My existence and interest in being a good partner for someone begs them to look past the stereotypes of disabilities. I want and need them to imagine what an alternate vision of a complete life might look like.

In my mind, being seen as worthy and valid through another person's eyes is a safer, happier place—and where I want to live. I wish I had always understood how important that was for me. This idea must have been rooted in my head since childhood as a result of the doctors being so adamant about me having to use legs so I could have a "normal" life and be accepted.

A few of my former girlfriends over the years shared some questions they received from friends about our relationship. They were asked things like "Did you know he didn't have any legs before you started going out with him?", "Did you stay with him after he had an accident?", "Was it a blind date and he didn't tell you about not having any legs?", and "Did you lose a bet?"

Given the negative stigmas and stereotypes associated with disability, able-bodied people who choose to interact with people who have disabilities are given additional moral credit for spending time with the disabled. This is often due to the perceived loss of social standing and potential in other people's eyes.

When my exes told their friends about my birth defect, they all reported receiving comments like "Good for you," "You're an amazing person," and "I wouldn't be able to do that."

My past partners also have been asked to answer insensitive or very specific questions about intimate things able-bodied people in a traditional relationship would never be asked.

Other people were inquisitive enough to want to know about how specific sexual positions work, possible deficiencies, and my personal favorite question, "Is it weird?"

My view is that everyone is allowed to share whatever parts of their life and the specifics of it with whomever they wish. However, I would ask people to be more self-aware of others' boundaries and to gauge within the context of the conversation what questions might not be appropriate. Or we can choose not to ask, to simply to respect other people's privacy. And, if someone chooses to self-disclose specifics, be all right with what they are willing to share unless given a green light to ask more detailed follow-up questions.

When asked personal questions about my physical relationships with partners, I always talk about how amazingly different every intimate relationship has been. No two people are ever the same. Some of the best parts of relationships have been finding out the unique things that people enjoy, then exploring how to be able to make each other happy in those ways.

The women I've dated were no better or worse than anyone else. They were women who took the time to get to know me to reap the benefits of being in a relationship with me. I have never believed that the particulars of any companionship needed to be broadcasted news.

Some of my most successful and longest relationships have been with women who told me, "You are the only person using a wheelchair I would ever date because you're not disabled." I think the reason they do not see me in that way is because I do not always see myself in that way.

When I am in a relationship, I aim to be what that other person needs me to be, and I do my best to meet their expectation. But sometimes it just isn't possible be-cause of my circumstances.

Like most people who date, I have been accepted and rejected by potential part-ners my entire life. When someone doesn't choose me back, the rejection hurts. Their excuses are pretty standard: "I just got out of a relationship and I'm not ready to com-mit to something or someone else," "You're gone traveling too much," or some form of the classic, "It's not you, it's me."

I understand where they are coming from. Working while traveling across the country without your partner is incredibly difficult. I found their reasons for rejection fine in the moment. In some cases, we happily became better friends. Because of those friendships, I would eventually learn the real reasons. Some of them confessed that my disability kept them from getting into a romantic relationship with me.

Stacy, a friend of mine, was trying to set me up with Alexa, one of her friends. Alexa told me she wasn't looking to date me and would rather just be friends. The next day, she texted Stacy asking, "Is Matt in a wheelchair?"

Alexa said that although it sounds awful, she can't even look at people in wheel-chairs. "My legs go numb and I've been known to fall down. I don't know if I can actu-ally agree to meet him at all."

Of the women who rejected me because of my disability, some were honest with me while others, like Alexa, were not. Of the honest ones, I was glad they came to me with their truth. It acknowledges the closeness, trust, and maturity of our relationships.

But it still hurts to know that my disability can be a romantic deal breaker for many people.

A movie I watched, *In the Company of Men*, sums up this idea perfectly. It tells the story of two men who makes a competition out of romantically pursuing a woman with a hearing impairment. At the end of the movie, she falls for the guy who stereo-typically is more attractive. But he was only playing her to win the bet.

She rejects the less attractive man who really had fallen in love with her. His feelings are hurt and, in a fit of rage, he tells her that because she has a disabling condition, she's not worthy to *choose* whom she falls in love with. He feels that she should be flattered that an ugly, able-bodied man would lower his standards enough to even consider dating a woman with a disability. He claims she should have known the attractive man must have been misleading her. Why else would he lower his social status by choosing to be with her?

In many people's minds, the presence of a disability automatically places me in one of society's underclasses. That movie and its message that I have internalized continue to serve as motivation for me to represent myself as able-bodied as I can. I want to be able to choose, too.

As I've said before, we really aren't that different, wheelchair or no wheelchair. I try to minimize my disability—and always have, in the hopes of people seeing me for who I am, not my wheelchair. Sometimes, though, that just isn't possible, especially when I'm interacting with people who aren't familiar with wheelchair users.

Years ago, I dated a girl from Russia. She emigrated here with her entire family when she was ten years old. It was awesome dating someone who had spent a great deal of her childhood living in another country. I would often ask her what it was like, and she would tell me stories about differences between the Russian and the American cultures.

One day, she asked if I would come with her to her father's birthday party. She said it was going to be at her house and that her entire family was going to be there. Their home was big and beautiful, but it was not accessible because it had a number of ornamental staircases located at the top of each entrance. It was the first time I had been invited there, so I had yet to develop a strategy for getting into their home.

To make matters worse, I wasn't told about the party until the day before because she "did not know how to have the conversation" with me.

"What conversation?" I asked.

"The conversation about you being on the floor of my parents' home."

Naively, I said, "What's the big deal about me being on the floor?"

That's when she averted her eyes from mine. "It is important to me that my parents never see you on the floor."

"Why?" I asked.

"When I told my parents I was dating a guy without legs, my dad asked, 'Why would you want to date a beggar?'"

I had been called many things before, but never a beggar. I think she could tell my feelings were hurt, so she immediately continued to tell me the rest of the conversation.

"I told him that you are *not* a beggar and that you are really successful and self-reliant."

I'll admit I was a little hurt, but that was trumped by my happiness as her comment showed that she cared about me. It showed me who she was.

Even though the father did not forbid her from seeing me, it was incredibly important to her that I never presented myself to her father on the floor, seen as a "beggar."

When I arrived to the party, we came in through a side entrance.

I carried my wheelchair up the stairs. I sat on the second step from the bottom and grabbed the front seat of the wheelchair with one of my hands. I faced away from the steps and used my other hand to help hike myself up to the third step and so on, all the while holding on to my chair while climbing up backward.

When I arrived at the top of the stairway, she and I met some of her cousins over the next few minutes, and we all entered the living room together. I made sure to never sit on the floor. I sat as tall as I could in my chair to limit my disability's visibility to her family. We all had a great time and the event went off without a hitch, except for when I pushed over to greet her father while he was sitting at the head of the kitchen table.

I met him on his right side and shook his hand with a smile. He didn't stand, which was fine. But later, my girlfriend told me he felt weird about not standing during the connection. She reported that he said later, "His chair was pushed in between the table and the wall, so there wasn't room to stand with his wheelchair there."

I could tell he was a bit put off in the moment. I thought it was because while I was sitting next to him in my tall wheelchair, my head towered over his by eight inches. I felt a strange power dynamic; he had to look up at me even though he was at the head of the table in his own home.

POINT TO PONDER: Have you ever had to represent yourself in a certain way to be acceptable to a significant other's family?

When I am in a relationship, I find myself using code switching and interpreting the idea a little more broadly. I use different words and phrases to express myself, I change my interests, modify my physicality and parts of myself to better align with the values and expectations of the person I am with. I do it to be more of a go-along get-along person, and to minimize the impact of my situation on the peripheral people in my partner's life.

It isn't the most comfortable thing for me to do. But if I can make my significant other's life easier when they are with me, I think it is the correct thing to do.

Years earlier, I was seeing a woman named Karen. Her birthday was coming up, and she said she had made plans to hang out with her friends.

I said, "That's cool. Do you think I could come along?"

She mentioned, "You'll have to talk to Cheryl; she's organizing the party."

I called Cheryl. "Karen told me you were putting something together for her birthday, and she said I should ask you if I could come along. Do you think that might be all right?"

She said, "I don't know if that's okay."

"Why wouldn't that be okay?"

Cheryl replied, "The party is at an indoor water park. We didn't know if you could do that, so we decided we wouldn't ask you."

Cheryl's fears of my feelings being hurt and her perception of something she assumed I couldn't participate in actually prevented her from inquiring about me possibly coming. It wasn't her job to protect me from myself. If she wanted to protect my feelings, a better way could have been by saying, "We were planning on it just being a girl's thing."

Over the phone, I told her, "Of course I can do water parks! I swim just fine and can leave my chair at the bottom of the slide and climb the stairs on my hands."

I ended up attending the party with her five best girlfriends and we all had a great day.

We spent time waiting on the steps of the waterslides, talking and carrying on. Our group spread out up and down the stairs. I would sit on the highest step as we moved toward the top of each waterslide. It provided me a little more height for the conversations and prevented me from always having to look eye level at her friends' butts. I guess that wasn't really so bad, though.

When you get below skin color, disabilities, and differences, at the very core of humanity, it's easy to see that we really aren't all that different. I just wish everyone else would see it that way, too.

I certainly don't want to leave the impression that it's impossible for me to find kind, considerate, and loving partners. In fact, I'd like to share with you the story about the best first date I ever had.

I met Candice at a convention, where I was immediately taken with her presence. When I found a good enough reason to initiate a conversation with her, I did so sheepishly because with her golden red hair, warm green eyes, and alluring smile, it was almost impossible for me to find words, even as a professional speaker.

We made good connections on a couple subjects and exchanged emails with the idea that we might be able to work together. After a few weeks, I reached out to get her input on a new project I was working on. She liked my musings and we both thought it would be a great idea if we got together to talk about it. On the day we agreed to meet, the weather was far too nice to be inside, and we decided to play hooky together.

We ended up going to an amusement park. I've always enjoyed riding roller coasters, but because of changing policies with insurance companies, I'm not always able to ride them. Most parks have a "three limb policy"—you have to have at least three real limbs, no type of prosthesis allowed. (I know this because once I packed one side of a pair of jeans with a hinged piece of wood, stuffed it with sweatshirts, and tied a shoe on the end. Needless to say, it didn't look real enough. But at least I tried.)

We went to Knoebels, an amusement park in central Pennsylvania with a variety of water and thrill rides along with roller coasters. It is known for having a one-of-a-kind trackless wooden coaster called the Flying Turns.

As Candice and I watched the bobsled on wheels swerve through the deep-valleyed wooden hairpin turns, I noticed it never went upside down. Although it didn't have a shoulder harness to hold me in, I thought I might be able to ride it safely because of the riders' seated position. Riders are seated two to a car, both facing forward, one in front of the other. A seat belt goes around the front rider, holding both people in and together. I imagined if she sat in front of me and wedged herself back into me, her body would serve as the best kind of safety restraint I have ever experienced.

I knew I needed to ride the Flying Turns with her, but I didn't know the park's policies, and I didn't want to have the conversation with her about the possibility of me not being able to ride due to my physical limitations. I understood how much she wanted to ride it as well.

I decided the best thing to do was to ask the security person by the ride's exit if I could go on. When I am allowed to ride, my party and I are allowed to go up the exit ramp, wait on the platform for a short while, and board the next train without waiting through the traditional line chain. It's a nice perk of Disability Privilege.

I yelled up to the gentleman, "Hey, do you think I can ride? I can transfer easily into the car."

He shook his head. "Not today. No wheelchairs on the platform. It's too busy."

I said back to him, "So on a different day when it isn't so busy, I could ride it?"

He nodded and said, "Yep!"

I felt cheated due to a subjective standard of "too busy." But there was a bit of a gray area he defined when he said no wheelchairs.

I motioned to get his attention again and asked, "If I could walk up the ramp I could ride?"

He said, "Yes."

That put me in a particular predicament. There was a way for me to ride with her, but it would force me to get out of my wheelchair, leave it unattended during the time it would take for me to walk up the 150-foot dirty wood ramp, wait to board, ride the ride, and walk back down to my chair—all on my hands without gloves...right after I saw a gentleman spit on the ramp where I'd have to walk.

For these reasons, I really didn't want to do it. It would put me in the position of being on the ground, and I didn't want her to have to see me like that or go through the embarrassment of being with me, a man crawling on the dirty walkway.

But I also knew that she heard the attendant say I could ride if I walked up the ramp. I didn't want to make the decision for both of us because I didn't want to start the day having to say no to riding, especially if that option was a possibility.

I turned to Candice. "I could get out of my wheelchair and walk on my hands up the ramp to the platform. Would that be okay?"

She said, "Sure."

I thought to myself, *All right but she has no idea what she's getting herself into.* If she was at all uncomfortable with me before, she had no idea how bad it was going to be when I was on the ground.

I jumped out of my chair, turned it upside down, and tried to put it far enough out of the way so people wouldn't mess with it. I started up the ramp. Luckily, I was wearing a pair of distressed jeans that got more distressed as I dragged them on the ground. I didn't bother to look back at her to see if she was following me. I tried to give her the chance to keep her distance if she didn't want to be part of this show. But by the time we got to the platform, she was standing behind me.

For safety reasons, roller coaster operators only want to have one person with a disability on the track at a time. That meant we had to wait an extended time before a car was ready for me. I sat on the burning hot imitation wood decking counting each of the trains as they were loaded. Group after group of riders worked their way to the boarding gates, waiting directly across from us. I could feel the weight of their stares. Some tried to redirect their eyes. But a forced obscured look away can be as hurtful to me as an opened-mouth gasp, coupled with a finger point directed at me.

Every three minutes, they all would get on their bobsled, and a new group of gawkers would take their place.

I tried to sit up straight and puff out my chest. Maybe it would help make people see me as something more than helpless. But then I realized that the zoo's alpha gorilla exerts its prowess in much the same way.

I was stuck in a bad place, and I could only hope that Candice wasn't feeling the angst and judgment that made me feel small. I didn't want to look up at her from the position of a child. I just sat there and waited for our turn to board the ride.

Then, I felt a hand grab mine. She had moved from standing behind me to sitting beside me. As I turned my head to notice, she leaned in and stole a kiss from me.

As I felt her soft lips meet mine, everyone and everything else disappeared. Instead of it being me against the world, she made it about us.

In that moment, by kissing me, she vouched for my validity. After the few seconds it took for me to recover from the best first kiss I've ever had, I took another glance across the tracks and saw that several of the couples who were spying on us before were now holding hands and smiling at each other.

Hers was the only acceptance I needed. She met me where I was, and I didn't even know I needed it until she gave it to me. She saw me in a situation where she thought she could help by making me feel included, making me feel like I belonged there and belonged with someone just like all the other couples on their journeys of love.

After we exited, I walked down the ramp and got back on my wheelchair. She leaned in, kissed me again, and said, "I hope it didn't bother you that I sat down with you on the platform. I just wanted to be close to you."

I grinned. "Anytime you want to hold my hand or kiss me, please be my guest."

"I hate to admit this," she said, "but part of me really enjoyed people watching us because I could show everyone how much I like you, and how much I appreciate being with you."

Before her kiss, I had made the situation all about me—how I was feeling, and how I was sure she must have felt too. But she was never uncomfortable. Those issues existed only in my mind, because of the insecurities I have about something I can't change.

Obviously, I need to be a better communicator and give people more of the benefit of the doubt when it comes to how they feel about being with me. I always try to hide the impact of my disability on other people, but sometimes it might be all right to share my burden.

Candice showed me the benefits of having an ally and an advocate in my life and what it could look like. Actually, she showed everybody. She gave me a gift I didn't know I needed at a time I would have thought that I couldn't have even accepted it. She stood up with me by sitting down.

POINT TO PONDER: How does acceptance of our situation change our outlook on life? Do we give up or press on with renewed purpose?

CHAPTER 2

I'm Not Disabled

A ll my life, I had one goal: not to be perceived as disabled. Life without legs was all I had known, and I felt as if I was getting by pretty well. I never understood why people looked at me and automatically assumed things about me—everything from how I manage to drive a car to the details of my sex life. I realized that others were putting limitations on me, and I didn't want that. I wanted to fit in and be normal—what *my* version of normal was.

In college, I started to play sports for the first time. I had always heard about wheelchair basketball and how awesome it could be. The coach of the wheelchair basketball team saw me and did his best to recruit me. He said he needed players who could play, and I needed to learn the skills to play. He tested my skill set by throwing basketballs at my head until I learned enough to catch them and not get hurt. This was his best attempt at combining the recognition of potential in players with a coach's tough love.

I got pretty good at catching, so I made the team. I wasn't great by any stretch of the imagination, but I had the qualifications: I owned a wheelchair, I had a disability, and I could catch a ball well enough.

In the sport of wheelchair basketball, everyone has some sort of permanent form of mobility impairment. It is a requirement to play. Disability is broken down into a very basic numeric system of ones, twos, and threes called "the classification system." The number you are assigned directly relates to your physical ability and level of disability. A "one" is typically a person who would be paralyzed from the chest down with no abdominal muscles or control of their lower extremities. A "two" usually has some abdominal muscles, but can't walk without the assistance of crutches or braces. Finally, a "three" is a person with a minimum disability, such as myself, without legs (or a leg), with a degenerative hip disorder or knee replacement surgery.

What is important to remember about the classification system and wheelchair sports in general is that everyone competing is the same in one way. As all players have "permanent" physical disabilities, we're essentially all on the same level. For many people with disabilities, sport is the only outlet they have to express themselves physically on a more equal basis against other people like themselves.

Unfortunately, though, one of the side effects of assigning defined point values based on a people's physical ability causes them to internalize and manifest their per-ceived value to the team. This can lead to one classification group making judgmental stereotypes about another one.

A player's point value determines an incredible number of things such as pref-erential seating in vehicles, how the delegation of responsibilities will be handed out, and social status (the pecking order) within a team. Many times, along with the as-signment of a lower classification number came the negative stigma that made certain players an easier butt of a joke or someone to lay blame upon.

At one point at the end of my competitive basketball experience, another player challenged my class three status. He claimed that my physical level of disability could actually qualify me to be "reclassified down" to a two.

If I had accepted the reassignment, it would have provided me more playing time and easier access to opportunities to play in international basketball competitions. I was unwilling to lose my social rank and the privileges that came with my assigned identity on the team, though. My status of being a "three" allowed me to internalize and claim my potential physical ability level to play wheelchair basketball very closely to a person who could walk with a minimum disability. If I started self-identifying as a "two," I assumed other players would think that I had hidden disabili-ties. They might ask, "What else is wrong with you?" Even within that community, I didn't want to be seen as someone potentially less than I had accepted myself as being.

Here I was playing on a wheelchair basketball team, yet I still sought to perceive myself from as far as disabled as possible.

Many times, though, it seems that my lifelong attempts to portray myself as just as able as everyone else are all for naught. Most frustrating is when this happens to me with friends.

A few years ago, I was Christmas shopping with one of my able-bodied friends, Greg. I was riding with him in his four-door Toyota Camry.

We pulled into the parking lot at the local Target store. He looked at me and said, "I only have a couple things to grab in there. Would you mind just waiting in the car for a minute while I run in, so I don't have to put your chair together and take it apart again?"

I totally understood what he was saying and, of course, I told him that was fine. I realize that able-bodied people stay in the car all the time, waiting for their friends just to run into a store. But my perception was that our relationship was being threatened by my inability to hide the extra work that sometimes comes along with my disability. The inconvenience of having to put together and take apart my wheelchair one more time served as a barrier to us spending more quality time together.

I didn't want to make him feel bad, so I didn't say anything. I thought, *for the rest of my life, people are probably going to make the easy decision of denying me opportuni-ties to be with them because it might take extra effort on their part.*

In order to keep my negative inner voice quiet and not have to deal with this scenario, I made a change in my life.

I decided to do everything I could to minimize the impact of my disability on the people around me. I would personally take care of as many of my specific needs as possible.

If I had to go somewhere with another person, I would drive them in my car. I wouldn't need them to take care of my wheelchair. If we were going to watch a movie at someone's house, I would invite everyone to my home, which is all on one level. I wouldn't have to crawl up the stairs or push through grass to enter through a basement door, making everyone around me feel bad for not having the perfect logistical accommodation for me.

Yes, taking on as many of my accommodations is more of a challenge. But it also makes me feel good, especially when the impact of my disability doesn't seem to be that big of a deal. Or when people say, "It is so easy to be with you."

Perfect.

POINT TO PONDER: In your relationships, do you find it easier to be the person people want or need you to be? How much of yourself are you willing to put aside to fit in with others?

CHAPTER 3

High Expectations

I have always set high expectations for myself. Why can't I do all the things that you can do just because I don't have legs? I refuse to acknowledge and empower my disability. Life is what we make of it.

When I was thirteen, my parents treated me like any other kid. They assigned to me certain chores around the house that I could do. Mostly, it was indoor jobs like cleaning my room, folding laundry, and emptying the garbage baskets around the house.

The outdoor jobs were my father's responsibility. He had a large, orange Simplicity riding mower that he would use on our lawn. I loved to watch him zoom around the yard. Sometimes, he would put me on his lap and let me steer while we mowed the lawn.

The older I got, the more I wanted to cut the lawn by myself. But not having legs is not ideal for operating a riding lawn mower brake pedal. I should mention the fact that this vehicle also has very sharp cutting blades attached. After a discussion with my father, he took the mower to the local machine shop and asked the owner to install a hand extension lever on top of the brake/clutch pedal. With that addition, it was now possible for me to completely control the machine, because the gas and speed were already controlled with a hand lever on the hood.

My father brought the mower home, taught me how to use all the levers, then sent me on my way to mow the lawn. Our house was on a large corner lot in town, with almost three quarters of an acre. The back yard was more uneven than the front, and we had a steep driveway. Most of my experience playing outside had been running on my hands, pulling or lifting myself around. All the while, I had to watch out for things in the yard like thistles, bees, small snakes, and sharp items.

The lawnmower gave me power over all of those threats. On the mower, I sat tall and I moved fast. It was a new mobility I hadn't felt before. The mower took me where I wanted to go on the property, all the while engaging in my favorite pastime: listening to music on my tape player and singing at the top of my lungs.

I was oblivious as to how entertaining this was for the people in our neighborhood. That is, until the day one of our neighbors asked my parents if I was available to mow their lawn. They explained how impressed they were with what I could do. My dad sent me over to handle the negotiation, and I was off on my way with my family's support and a little bit of Disability Privilege. After the neighbor saw that I was capable and dependable, I decided to approach a few other neighbors. The summer mowing business became a lucrative job for me.

This was my first job, and by keeping this mindset, I figured I could have just as "normal" of a work life as everybody else, and I did. In addition to my weekend disc jockey business in high school and through college, I delivered oxygen bottles to home care patients and fixed their wheelchairs, bath benches, and walkers for a medical supply company.

By the time I finished college with a Bachelor of Science degree in communication and a minor in history, I was a decent wheelchair basketball player and had also developed a business relationship with an Australian sport wheelchair manufacturer named Mogo Wheelchairs.

I started designing and distributing wheelchairs for elite-level athletes affiliated with different sports throughout North America. With this background, I figured that I would be qualified for a bunch of jobs in the medical supply industry. But I fell into thinking as many young people do: What do I want to do for a career? I had *no* idea if working those kinds of jobs would make me happy for the long term or what I should thinking about doing instead.

My father told me I should look into having a "headhunter" help me find a job. He explained how it was their job to assist specialized people to find jobs appropriate for them based on their skill sets.

I printed out a list of fifteen headhunters in the Milwaukee area and decided to drive to each office and hand them a copy of my résumé. I woke up early the next morning and dressed in the business suit I received as a graduation present from my father. It was a typical day in the middle of snowy December so driving was extremely slow, not to mention how hard it is to push a wheelchair through inches of snow and ice.

I found myself leaving phone messages for people and sliding my résumé under doors all day. A few times, I was able to speak to someone in the office. They would attempt to sell me on the jobs they had to offer. Some of the jobs included selling floor mats to companies or managing the cardboard, honor-coded candy vending systems for offices.

They would explain how lucrative the job could be for a hard worker. But then they would start speaking a little slower when they explained the part of the job that entailed carrying around lots of merchandise. While everyone was nice to assure they would keep me in mind for the next opportunity, I was a bit down on the way this process was playing out.

It was almost the end of the day, and I was down to the last name and address on my list. Luckily, it was a commercial building about ten minutes away. It had just started snowing again, and I was cold. I got back into my car and began the short drive. The suite number read 323 on the sheet of paper—that meant it would be on the third floor. I also knew because of the classification of real estate, there would likely not be an elevator.

When I arrived, I recognized the building. I could see the staircase through the front door window. The door was propped open with snow from people opening it all day. The office manager had neglected to shovel the walk, stoop, or landing.

I could have easily given up that day, but something inside pushed me to keep going. I think I believed that the harder I worked for something, the better it would pay off for me. I grabbed my briefcase and wheelchair and was off.

I opened the front door and moved toward the flight of stairs I had to climb. Each stair felt like it had the cool rigidity of cement under it, and an all-weather rubber coat-ing was glued to its sides. To prevent an able-bodied person's shoe from slipping off each step, it had an industrial sandpaper strip two inches wide running the width of each step. The sharp pieces of grit grabbed and pulled at the wet, thin cotton material of my pants as I sat on the edge of each step and dragged myself over it.

The rest of the rubber coating had just enough of a moat to hold the dirty water remnants of the snow as each stranger's dirty shoes and boots released the debris throughout the day. My pants were new and clean on the first step. But by the fifth step, I could no longer say the same.

As I approached the third floor at least the steps were dry. But I was tired and felt the weight of the day in my shoulders. I couldn't stop, though. I knew the only thing I had to look forward to was claiming the path I had just dredged through, like planting a flag on Mt. Everest. That's just what I had to do.

I soldiered on, and as I reached the last landing on the third floor, I saw a woman locking the door of an office I judged to be near suite 323.
I called out to her, "Beth?"

I knew I had made an appointment with her close to the end of the day. She was closing up, and I hated to think she had given up on me. She replied, "Matt?"

I said, "Yes, please just give me a moment to collect myself and I will be right there."

She proceeded to reopen her door and went back inside. I stabilized my chair, lifted myself back on it from my position on the floor, folded the wet and grimy por-tions of my pants under my legs to hide the mess, and grabbed my bag and moved down the hallway to see her.

It was a short meeting because of the time of day, but an overall much better experience. The first thing she said to me was "I wish you would have told me you were in a wheelchair. I would have offered to meet with you at the McDonald's down the street."

I have been to many meetings with strangers who were interested in accommodating my disability. I guess people know that McDonald's are accessible. I didn't want to tell her about not having legs, because I didn't want her to pre-judge me before I had the chance to show her all the things I could do.

After looking over my résumé, she asked, "With so many things listed on your résumé that you are currently doing, how would you have any time to do another full-time job?"

I responded, "Most of the things I do are on the weekends or things I can do in my spare time. I'd really like to have an opportunity to work in a corporate environment from nine to five."

She opened her leather attaché case and pulled out a piece of paper. "I have one opportunity with a small Fortune 50 company, but I don't know if it's the right fit. The person for this position needs to have a corporate sales background. I can see that you have some small sales experience, but I don't know if that's enough."

I explained a little more about how I sold my wheelchairs and marketed my disk jockey service. She said, "I'll put your name forward and we'll see if they bite."

As we left her office, I knew that I was going to have to carry my wheelchair back down all the steps. She offered to help, but I declined. She could have walked down the stairs faster, but she stalled and waited with me as I struggled with my chair.

At the bottom of the stairwell, just before we ventured outside, she grabbed my hand and said, "From what I have already seen, I know you can do the job. If you are willing to put that much effort into just reaching me, I'm sure you'll be able to sell to and manage a customer base. It was really great meeting you. You will hear from me soon."

CHAPTER 4

Best Intentions

B eth phoned me less than a week later and helped me get placed at a job where I focused on selling telecommunication equipment to small and medium-sized companies. Linda was one of my first managers, and she was also the person I felt closest to at the company.

She was stationed out of the Minneapolis office, but she traveled extensively around the Midwest. Linda's energy for the job and her enthusiasm for developing new talent made her ideal for the offices that needed more direction, like ours.

What made her so special was that she was tough when she needed to be, but she was also very fair. Linda always seemed to have the right answer for everything. It was truly magical to witness.

Unfortunately, her incredible work ethic and track record of success also brought with it some jealousy. There were some people in the company who didn't appreciate her. They couldn't attack her for the quality of how she did her job; the only thing they could use to disparage her was, in their minds, her personal life.

Linda was a lesbian, and she engaged in an alternative lifestyle compared to most of the other people in the office. However, just like all the other salespeople, Linda would share stories around the watercooler about what she did with her partner over the weekend. But because of the same-sex nature of her relationship with the love of her life, the straight members of our team would say things behind her back like "I don't know why she always has to be talking about it and throwing her lesbian relationship in our faces." Or they would make even cruder comments about the potential nature of their intimacy.

All the things they said really bothered me because I didn't like to hear people undermine her "lifestyle." So, I never engaged in that talk and chose to leave the room when people would undermine her.

I never thought anything bad about her relationship. I even believe that it was Linda's personal experience that gave her such incredible insight on how to overcome adversity and how to motivate people. She was a living, breathing example of what everyone should attempt to be.

All the negative talk about her went on for over a year, and I had finally had enough. I needed to speak up and take action.

I went to talk to her.

I didn't want people saying things behind her back. I thought that if she could just fit into the corporate culture in Wisconsin a little bit better, she could have even more success. I truly thought I was going to help Linda, but it turns out I was wrong.

I picked the moment to speak with her when we were working at a job fair together. I thought I had enough credibility in our relationship to talk to her about what was being said behind her back.

We were eating lunch at a small table in the back of the conference center. I asked her, "Is it okay if I tell you something that bothers me that is happening in the office?"

She nodded, listening.

I began, "Other salespeople in the office are bothered by you always talking about your partner. They feel like you're pushing your alternative lifestyle on them. I think you would do better if you just toned it down a little when you were in the office." I told her, "If you would just keep your stories a little closer to your vest, you would be more respected at the office and not ridiculed behind your back as much."

I thought I was trying to help a friend, but in reality, I was asking her to minimize her life and her loving relationship with her partner—all the while telling her to try to be someone else, so she could be more successful with people who didn't want to be her friend or work with her anyway, and so I would feel better about the disparaging office gossip.

I was worse than her co-workers because I discriminated against her to her face. In three minutes of conversation, I destroyed a valued friendship.

I didn't expect what happened next. Linda became so upset that she left the job fair. I tried to apologize, but I had no idea what made her so distraught. I couldn't imagine how what I said could have elicited such a response, and from someone to whom I felt so close. I tried to follow her and to make things better, but to no avail.

The following morning, I received a phone call from Linda, requesting that I meet her for breakfast. She explained that we needed to have a very serious conversation that morning if we ever hoped to maintain any kind of a relationship.

We met in the hotel restaurant. She was already seated as I joined her. I immediately began trying to say I was sorry for what happened. My apologies for what hurt her feelings became apologies for my lack of understanding of the importance and significance of the situation.

Linda began to explain by telling me a story about what actually happened behind the scenes during the last interview before I was hired by this company. The three top regional managers in the company conducted my final interview, and Linda was one of those managers. The interview consisted of a thirty-minute presentation that I needed to make about something I felt really passionate about. I chose to do my presentation on the value of integrating wheelchair sports into the mainstream K-12 public school gym class curriculum. I brought wheelchairs to demonstrate different sports, and I wore my basketball uniform for the program. Each of the managers participated in short simulations, and I felt like I knocked it out of the park. My feelings were confirmed by the position being offered to me, and my acceptance of their offer.

However, the story that Linda shared with me about my hiring process was much different. After my third interview, all three managers agreed that I seemed to be a great person with fine energy. But both of the men had genuine reservations about my ability to do my job because of the nature of my disability.

Neither one of them thought I would be able to keep up with the workload, handle the cold calling on businesses, or be able to do the physicality of toting the products. They raised serious questions about my overall health and how the changes in weather could affect my job performance. They even wondered if the market would be accepting of someone with a disability. They felt that business owners might not be "comfortable" with a person with a disability in their shop.

In order to be hired, all three of the managers had to agree. Only Linda served as my advocate in the meeting. She took it upon herself to educate the other two managers about what I could do and what I could bring to the business and to my customers. It was Linda who convinced the other managers that I had the potential and the ability. She stood up for me when I couldn't stand up for myself.

She didn't feel like I should downplay or dismiss the fact that I had a disability. She explained to the managers that it wasn't going to keep me from being able to do my responsibilities. She worked hard to convince the other two men that I could do the job.

That's when the reality of what I had done hit me in the head like a falling piano from a cartoon. What hurt her the most was when I had the opportunity to be her advocate, I did not stand up for her. I didn't stand up to the salesmen who were belittling her and the relationship she had with her partner. Instead, I chose to do the opposite. I was asking her to stop telling people about who she actually was. It was even more selfish on my part because I wanted Linda to stay "in her closet" so my feelings wouldn't be hurt when I heard the other salesmen talking about her.

I should have stepped up and told the team that what they were saying was not only inappropriate and had the capacity to get them all fired, but that it was hurtful because they relied on their grossly ignorant feelings and their fear of the unknown to tear down the most honest and genuine person in the office.

I wish I had understood and could articulate then what I know now, because during the next few days after I talked to her, I just kept thinking about it. *How could I have been so blind? How could I have not understood why she reacted the way she did?*

I acted inappropriately to a person I valued as a friend.

Linda never once asked me to tone down my difference by wearing prosthetics, covering my legs, or engaging in any other minimizing behavior. Now I understand why it was so damaging to her and how my previous words and actions undermined my friendship with her. I vowed that I would never do it again.

I tried to rebuild our relationship the best I could, but Linda was soon reassigned to manage another team back in Minnesota. The time I had hoped to spend with her to rebuild the relationship never materialized. This was one of the hardest lessons I have ever learned.

POINT TO PONDER: Have you ever acted inappropriately in a way that destroyed a friendship? Did you have a chance to apologize to make things right—and did you take it?

During my seminars, people often come up to me and tell me they love my enthusiasm and my never-give-up attitude. It's ingrained in me. And, a big surge of my being able to keep up that energy is by the friends I surround myself with.

Have you ever met someone before and you could see their spirit in their eyes? I call those people "bright eyes." They are the type of person you can walk up to and have a conversation that leaves you wanting to spend more time with them. That describes my friend James. When I first met him, I could see his light right away. His energy lifted hearts and brought smiles to everyone within earshot. His sense of humor resembled my own, and I knew this was someone I wanted to spend more time with.

James and I were taking a day trip into Canada. As a country they do not have a legal set of requirements that guarantee me access to most places like they do in the US. I didn't really want to have to tell James that I might need his help, and that there might be some things we couldn't do.

When this happens, I make sure to let whomever I am with know that I will just stay back. I always suggest that they should just do whatever it is without me. When they do make the choice to not participate, I feel guilty for preventing them from having their able-bodied experience. This is especially true when I'm with a new friend. I don't want my disability to prevent them from experiencing their abilities fully. If I perceive that as happening, it places more emphasis on my disability in my mind, which undermines my confidence.

I cautiously mentioned to James that Canada doesn't have the ADA, so I might need a hand up or a potential wheelchair carry. Without missing a beat, he mentioned that he used to take care of his grandfather who was in a wheelchair for many years. James said he would gladly do whatever I needed. It was a meaningful moment for me. Not only did he alleviate my insecurity, but he also revealed a part of his life to me.

When I spend time with people who have had previous experiences with people who have disabilities, more times than not, I find myself able to develop connections with them faster. They are not merely fascinated with the novelty of disability. They understand how to be a person's advocate within the framework of Disability Privilege.

I have seen people make real changes in themselves after they have cared for someone else. Whether it is a newfound empathy for someone's living condition, or a college student assisting in rebuilding a house for someone who lost their home to a weather-related tragedy. Those hours affect people.

CHAPTER 5

All The Things I Cannot Do

W ait, there are *some* things I can't do because I'm disabled. But I'm learning to be okay with it.

Not having legs *does* make me truly disabled. It prevents me from being able to push my car out of a snowbank. If I had a family and our home was on fire, I wouldn't be able to grab each one of my kids under my arms and run out to save their lives. Not having legs kept me from being able to join the military and fight for my country after 9/11.

In addition to knowing all the physical things I can't do, the absence of my legs prevents me from having some typically desirable, able-bodied experiences with another able-bodied person—like holding hands with someone while walking with them.

My inability to achieve moments like that one stirs the most damaging insecurity I have: not knowing how the manifestation of my disability will keep me from being "enough" for someone else. My biggest fear has always been appearing to be less than desirable, especially to a romantic partner.

Another one of my ex-girlfriends showed me how that felt when she sent me a picture postcard of her ice skating with her new boyfriend. While we dated, I noticed Angelica loved the winter and always kept a pair of ice skates hanging on the wall of her coat closet. When we first got together she asked, "Can you go ice skating?"

I told her about when I was younger and had a welder friend of mine weld ice skates to a skateboard in place of the wheels. Then I took it out to a local ice arena to try it, and as I sat on it and pushed around on the ice with my hands, the manager of the rink ran out and said, "You can't use that!" He claimed the sharp blades on other people's skates would cut my fingers off.

Apparently ice skating with her boyfriend was more important to Angelica than I thought, because after our hard breakup she sent the postcard to me and drew a large smiley face on the back. The photograph and note worked nicely to reinforce that worry in my relationships.

My insecurities about my inabilities never drive my feelings when I'm alone, however. I feel complete and fully capable when I'm driving my car or functioning in my own home. I've created those places to be perfect environments for me. Everything is accessible. I require no regular help from anyone. The things I don't do or can't do are things I chose not to do or even care about—like using the top shelf in the kitchen cabinets or hanging Christmas lights on tall trees outside. When I'm by myself, I don't have to worry about disappointing someone, because I don't have to worry about meeting their needs or expectations.

POINT TO PONDER: Should I be concerned about being "enough" for others? Do you have that same fear?

When I'm traveling with other disabled people on competitive sports teams, there are always able-bodied people around with the assigned job of taking care of our general needs. Just a few of the many things they handle are putting our wheelchairs together for us while we get in and out of vehicles. It's their responsibility to carry our team's gear and manage all the logistics of housing and transportation. As a result, I find it easier to be more confident in public because I don't feel an obligation to manage everything for myself, making sure my disability isn't negatively impacting the able-bodied people around me.

From 1997 through 2004, I served and participated as a member of the United States Paralympic Sitting-Volleyball Team. I played in the Paralympic Games in Sydney, Australia and served as the first alternate for the games in Athens in 2004.

Some people today still confuse the Special Olympics with the Paralympic Games. The Special Olympics is the world's largest sports organization for children and adults with intellectual disabilities, providing year-round training and competitions to more than 4.4 million athletes in 170 countries.

The Paralympic Games is the second largest competitive sports competition in the world. The games are played every four years directly after the Olympics, and in the same venues and facilities. All of the athletes have some kind of qualifying physical disability. In the US all of our athletes have the same status and responsibilities as able-bodied Olympic athletes; we are held to the same standards regarding drug abstinence and acceptable behavior.

The Paralympics are organized in tandem with the Olympic games. The derivation of the name is often wrongly confused and assumed to represent "paralyzed" people, instead of the proper representation of competing in "parallel to" the Olympic games, hence "Paralympics."

Even though Team USA came to the Sydney games well prepared, we knew that we were in for a heck of a ride. Within the boundaries of North and South America, we did very well. With US support, we trained alongside the able-bodied athletes at the Olympic Training facility in Colorado Springs, Colorado.

Quite simply, our team's challenge was the talent pool was drawn from a relatively small group of US Americans. Up to the early 2000s, we didn't have many victims of land-mines or IEDs, which unfortunately "assist" other countries with their Paralympic recruiting. I know that sounds rough, crude, and heartless, but it's the truth.

From my experience it seems like countries such as Iraq, Iran, and Bosnia at that time all had very strong and famous Paralympic teams as a result of the war-torn reali-ties of their environments: land-mines, wars, and atrocities. The countries had to be very inclusive in how they integrated their children who were disabled. The high ratios of students with disabilities to teachers forced mainstreaming and inclusion in their schools.

Many countries have far superior Paralympic teams and a wider acceptance of wheelchair sports as mainstream because of the high numbers of able-bodied and people with disabilities playing and competing against each other. These countries have very strong talent pools from which to draw national team players.

We knew that the best teams from around the world would probably remain the top teams, even at the Paralympic Games. However, that didn't stop us from training as hard as we could or preparing for the games by taking advantage of all the other resources we had available to us, such as facilities, strength and conditioning, nutrition, etc. The reality, however, was that our gold medal dreams were dashed, as we ended up being defeated during the initial rounds of competition.

That was when I decided it was now up to me to have my own "gold medal experience." I wanted to have something that no one else could claim to have accomplished during the games. I was determined that my disability would not present any special challenges for me in accomplishing this crowning achievement.

If you ever travel to the city of Sydney, Australia, there are a couple of things you should know. First, it is a great and beautiful city. If you are willing to endure the flight, it is worth your time to see the harbor and, of course, the Sydney Opera House and the Sydney Harbor Bridge.

While I was there, I heard that it was possible to climb the Sydney Harbor Bridge. You could start at one sidewalk, climb up the supports to the top, then come back down the other side. It seems that a businessman saw an op-portunity and asked the city if he could lease the area above the bridge. They said yes, and his bridge climbing tour experience was born.

I asked someone if any double amputee Paralympic athlete had climbed the bridge. The typical climb involves ascending 465 steps made of aluminum grating that transport you to the highest point in the center of the bridge, 134 meters above Sydney Harbor. Then, you descend the same side. It's not exactly wheelchair accessible. It seemed as though, up until my brilliant idea, no one like me had even dared to try it.

This became my mission—I would climb the bridge. I mean, how hard could it really be? I originally was going to do it with a friend of mine on the team. However, much to my disappointment on the morning of the last day when I looked for him, we kept missing each other. I decided to attempt the imposing feat with a woman I met during the games.

We set off for the attraction and were initially stymied by the inconvenient location of the ticket booth. We thought it might be close to the bridge and we could buy our tickets there. No such luck. We found out that the ticketing center was a few blocks away from the bridge. We also found one more potential obstacle: The ticketing center was located on an elevated floor in a building with no handicapped-accessible entrance. Justifying this, I thought to myself, *Why should it be handicapped accessible? The experience itself is not. This type of challenge never stopped me from stepping up to my challenges in the past.*

When we arrived at the ticketing center, I carried my wheelchair up the stairs. We approached the counter to purchase our tickets. I was met with looks of amazement and confusion. I offered my converted currency to the ticket seller, explained to her that I wanted to climb the bridge. I was refused tickets on the grounds that it couldn't be done because of my wheelchair.

I tried to explain to her that I wouldn't be using the wheelchair to make the climb; I would be doing it on my hands. With a look of amazement, she still persisted and said it wasn't available to me. I remained calm and asked to speak to a manager or someone of higher authority.

The next fellow took me aside and explained that it was not just the steps that he saw as a barrier to my engaging in the experience. While on the bridge, everyone had to wear a gray jumpsuit to blend in, so as not to distract people driving on the bridge. To make matters even more complicated, everyone ascending the bridge is tied to the hand-railing with a harness to keep them from jumping or falling off the side. Tethers from the harness are tied onto the waists of participants and then tied to the bridge. The tether positioned at the hip level is fine for someone who is walking. But for someone like me who would be climbing on their hands, the harness and tether would fashion itself into a noose.

I sized up the situation and came up with the idea that I could wear the gray jumpsuit, but with the leg bottoms tucked into the waist belt. My pants would serve as a cushion and provide me a bit more protection. The challenge of belts and harness would be overcome if I could tie it all together and cinch them around my legs. This would give the length and flexibility I needed. I explained all of this to the manager in charge. Yet he claimed that even with my plans and modifications, it was still a no go.

I have never really been one to look for help in places and situations where I thought I could get the job done myself. But from time to time, I must admit, I do need help from outside sources. This was one of those times.

Being a Paralympic athlete is a great honor and it comes with a number of respon-sibilities. One of those responsibilities is to represent yourself and the United States in a positive and professional manner while on the team in competition, when traveling, and in your everyday life. Team members go through extensive training involving eti-quette, behavior, and media interaction. We were told, "Everyone is always looking for a story. Always keep that in mind and make our country proud."

I wanted to make our country proud, so I alerted the media in Sydney to this amazing, wonderful opportunity I would be pursuing. What I didn't explain to them was that I was forbidden to actually make the momentous trek. Oh, what a tangled web we weave…

When I arrived back at the Sydney Harbor Bridge about an hour later with camera crews and the local media present, the story was now a little different. I explained to the manager what a great honor it was to be able to do this during this special time of the games. I shared how this huge physical barrier was going to be overcome by a person with a disability for the first time in history. And finally, I hyped what a great story it would be to promote his tour business and his progressive thinking toward what people can achieve if they put their mind to it.

With the media spotlight, how could they refuse? They didn't. They offered a spe-cial guided tour for myself and my companion, and we made our way to the bridge, along with the media.

All I wanted to do was climb the bridge. However, sometimes I choose not to do or am kept from doing something for good reasons.

At one point when I was younger, I wanted to go on a tandem skydive out of an airplane. The gentleman who was assisting me in the jump thought it would probably be fine, but he couldn't completely guarantee my safety. Needless to say, you only get one chance to see if the harness works. I put that one on the shelf.

But I really thought I had thoroughly worked through this problem with climbing the bridge. It turns out, I hadn't. I was in denial: I allowed my desire for the outcome to supersede common sense. I am not invincible.

First of all, I left my wheelchair at the ticket office and decided to make my way to the bridge on my hands. I had no idea that the bridge climb entrance was several blocks away from the ticket office. Every day, I lift my body up with my arms and throw myself forward while rocking to maintain the inertia of the movement. Basically, I am lifting my body weight up and moving forward about a foot and a half. I don't spend that much of my time on the floor. So, to do this to cover the distance to the bridge took the wind out of me before we even got there.

I started to feel the same pressure the bridge manager felt. Now, I started to wonder if I was even going to make it to the bridge. I sized up my three motivating factors: I wanted to beat the bridge, I wanted to impress my new female companion, and finally, I wanted the media to witness and document my accomplishment.

Soon we made it to the bridge. We then had to climb through the support of the bridge to get to the stairs. Oh, yes—the stairs. They were not the typical stairs people would have in their house or something you would find in a public building. They were the kind of textured metal steps made out of the grating material that cleans your muddy boots or shoes off as you are climbing the stairs. It's perfect for providing a safe and secure step for walking on. But the sharp edges were hard on my hands and bottom. It all added to my personal challenge.

I started climbing, and it was hard. Not only was the physicality intense, but I was also now confronting another fear that I didn't even know I had: the big fear of heights! I would imagine that my years of general proximity to the ground helped me develop my love for being close to the earth. I tried to rely on "don't look down" thinking. But looking at the next step required a good glance down through the metal barricades and support girders.

With pride and persistence, we reached the top. I was a bit tired—actually, I was exhausted! My hands looked as if they had been through the war. The metal grating took the first and second layers of calluses off my hands, which had been toughened over the years. I had twisted from side to side on my buttocks to uncover different angles and positions that helped me resist the barbs on the steps. The pant legs of the gray jumpsuit had worn through my denim jeans underneath, and I was just halfway there. That's right—the top isn't the top—it's just halfway. What goes up must come down.

I remembered some of the movies I had seen about people climbing Mount Everest. Many times, climbers reach the summit but never make it down to revel in their accomplishment. I was determined that this wasn't going to happen to me.

Because I had set such a high expectation for myself by bringing along a companion—and not to mention the media—I knew I could not give up now. I was beginning to have real problems with my hands, and I shared that with our guide. He proceeded to offer up a pair of gloves he had in his pocket that he sometimes used when it was chilly. I put them on and mercifully found my salvation. It was the last tool I needed to accomplish my mission.

We climbed back down the stairs, through the supports, and back to the ticketing center. Someone had brought my wheelchair to the bottom of the bridge for me—a welcome sight.

When we arrived at the ticketing center, there was quite a celebration. The media got their story, the bridge got their promotion, and I got my "gold medal" experience. The bridge organization offered me the honor of placing my picture on the wall recognizing those hardy souls who have climbed the bridge before me. They asked me to sign it. I wrote, "Taking life one step at a time."

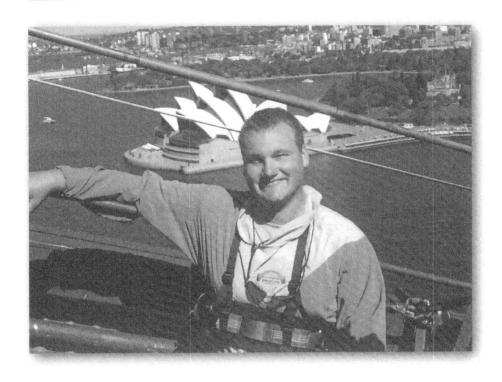

CHAPTER 6

The ADA

After turning forty, I came to the realization that I have effectively lived two different lives: one as a disabled person before I graduated high school in 1991 and one as an almost able-bodied person since then.

I am not saying that I was "healed" of my birth defect on my eighteenth birthday. Nor was I spared the quiet sting of not being able to participate in something because of insurance regulations and limitations. For the most part, I have had the privilege of knowing what it feels like to go from "not having access" to public places, activities, and events to being able to have an "assumption of access" just like able-bodied people. I do not have to live my life like a second-class citizen.

Before I started using the wheelchair in high school, while I was still walking with prosthetics, my family's day-to-day life revolved around finding the right kind of public and private restrooms I could use. Every place we went, we needed a large enough bathroom stall or open space to accommodate my taking the legs on and off to relieve myself.

I would have to repeat this process time and time again in public bathrooms at baseball stadiums, gas stations, restaurants, schools, malls, hotels, churches, and national parks. Physically having to lay down in filth, snow, feces, grease, and urine was part of my life.

When a better accommodation was present, it was generally developed out of the "charity" model. It required a firsthand experience the business owner had with a family member or a friend who needed it. I was forced to rely on people's goodwill and on their understanding of other people's needs, based on their own personal experience. It was very limiting and without the established standards for general accommodations, the inconsistencies were almost as disabling as there not being any accommodations at all.

After I graduated from high school, I started to have an expectation of accessibility within the places I wanted to go. As a country, we have been steadily moving toward that as a reality. Those changes occurred because of the passage of a 1990 law called The Americans with Disabilities Act.

The ADA was the crown jewel in the efforts of an entire generation of people who fought for my right to have equal access to public places before I ever knew I needed them. The legislation allows me to have the same expectation of general access to the same or similar experiences as most able-bodied people.

It also helps to provide and define a specific framework of guidelines, policies, and standards for what proper accessibility should look like. In public places, for example, round doorknobs are no longer legal; they must be a flat rotating handle that can be pushed down or up to open the door. Alternatively, the mechanism must be a straight bar that when pushed forward, lifts the latch and allows the door to open. This is because a person without the full use of their hands might not be able to grip a round doorknob to open the door in the event of a fire.

Before the ADA, the front side of public drinking fountains used to run straight down from the edge of the bowl to the ground. Now the law states that the drinking fountains must have enough space under them to accommodate the front foot space of a wheelchair to give the user the ability to get close enough to position themselves over the spout to get a drink.

Door close buttons on many elevators don't respond when pushed because the ADA states that the doors have to stay open for at least three seconds after the last motion sensor in the doors are triggered. This is intended to give people who might move a little slower a better chance to not to get hit by the closing doors.

Many years of work, discussion and the negotiation and passage of the ADA ultimately gave me access to a higher quality of life in our country. I have witnessed first-hand, how it has literally given new life to people with disabilities by granting them access and privilege. The ADA has given me the ability to live as normally as I can, just like everyone else.

My life before the ADA was drastically different. When I had the ability to use the wheelchair in school for that short time, there were still challenges. I couldn't fit into the school bathroom stalls because they were too narrow. I would have to jump out of the wheelchair onto the floor in front of the toilet on my hands and bottom, then proceed to pull myself on top of the toilet bowl and seat. But it was still better than the procedure for using the restroom with the prosthesis. The only way to do that was to hold on to one crutch and set the other one on the floor. With my free hand, I would bend over and grab the toilet bowl and lean backward on the crutch to release the lock mechanism in the knee. I would do my best to manage a controlled forward fall to the floor on the wooden knees of the prosthetics. Then, I would lie down sideways on the floor and swing the legs around under the bowl so I could lie down with my back against the floor, straddling the toilet between my prosthetic legs. I had to be in that position to unbuckle the belt and to pull my pelvis and little legs out of the limbs. Finally, I would take off my pants and crawl over the legs and lift myself onto the toilet and use it. Reversing the process finished the job. If you are exhausted just picturing this procedure, imagine living it on a daily basis four or five times a day.

Today, handicapped- and wheelchair-accessible stalls are required in every establishment's bathroom. You never realize the importance of this until you have to crawl on the floor to use the toilet, especially in an elementary school. I've noticed improvements in elementary school bathrooms over the years, especially since I visit elementary schools a few times per year for speaking engagements.

My favorite part about these speaking engagements is listening to questions from students. Most times, students' questions are great and but pretty basic, because they are just trying to figure out what they like and what works for them. Their newfound personal preferences are perfect subject matters for them to draw on when they are trying to connect with someone new. Many times the first question they ask me is simply, "What is your favorite color?"

I immediately reply with a question of my own. "Well, what is *your* favorite color?"

They quickly respond with the name of their color. No matter what they tell me, I always say, "That's my favorite color, too!" Okay, it's a little white lie. But, establishing my favorite color is less important than trying to relate to them.

Once we've established relatability, it becomes easier to talk about what other things we have in common. I use this as a first step to make them see me as more like them than not.

But if you want to know my real favorite color, it is blue—reflex blue, to be specific: the color blue often associated with the handicapped symbol. When I see that color blue on a sign publicly displayed, I know that someone was thinking about how to make my life easier.

If I try to look at things from an able-bodied perspective, I'm surprised that everyone isn't more appreciative for the way things are put together for them. Stairs and steps function quite well. Twenty-two to twenty-eight-inch-wide doors on public restrooms work well for most people. These are things most people simply take for granted. It's all part of the "privilege" that able-bodied people have, and they don't even know it.

All I'm trying to do is to live my life in an able-bodied world and fit into their architecture, their design. Even though I'm trying to fit in and act as if I don't need anyone's help, the reality is that I'm looking for all the clues and considerations I can find to make my life easier. When I see my blue, I recognize that as the color of handicapped accessibility.

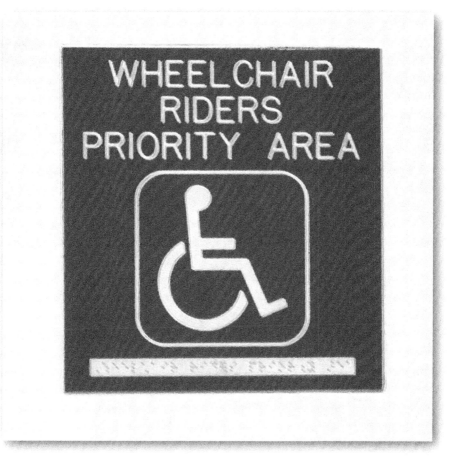

I understand that most able-bodied people might not even notice these inconspicuous signs. The signs don't mean anything special to a person until they need them.

When I see those blue signs, I say to myself, "Look how cool this is! My advance team was here and they left me bread crumbs to know where to go."

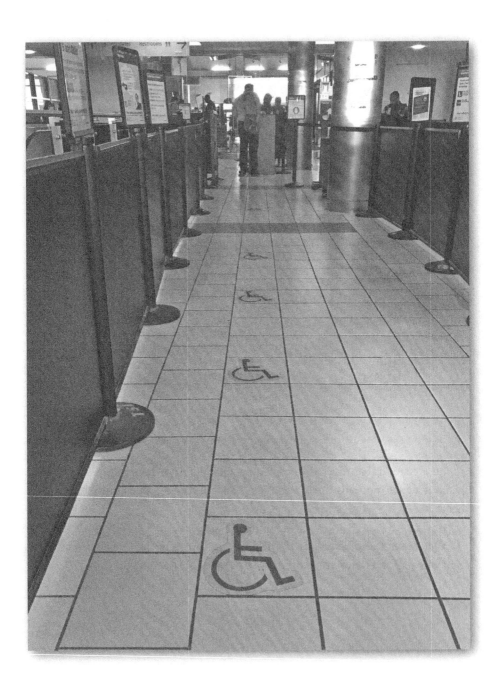

I know I'm not alone in finding comfort in this directed signage. There are thousands of posts and directional markers for helping people. Around towns in America, there are often large signs that welcome the public to local communities by listing the badges or banners of the local service clubs. People indicate interests and memberships in organizations through waving flags and displaying signage. People like to know they belong. The color blue activates those feelings in me.

I lived the first twenty years of my life being my own advance team. I was both Lewis and Clark. I invested plenty of time and effort into crawling and making my way through mazes just to be shown at the last corner that I wasn't capable of finishing my journey. When I see reflex blue, it means someone has blazed a trail for me; it is comforting to know that my day just got a little easier.

In recent years, the ADA and everything it stands for has changed for the better: As a society, we are making progress. I particularly like the evolution of the visual representation of the "universal disabled person." Most people are familiar with the symbol. Just in case you are not, it's the stick figure side-view of a person in a wheelchair. All handicapped parking signs display it in some form.

A few years ago, I started to see different interpretations and examples of the wheelchair person graphic appear on signage. There are a few manifestations of the rebranding of the design. I found the one I like the best when visiting New York's Museum of Modern Art. It is called The Accessible Icon Project. Tim Ferguson Sauder, Brian Glenney, Sara Hendren, and the team at Triangle, Inc. created the image.

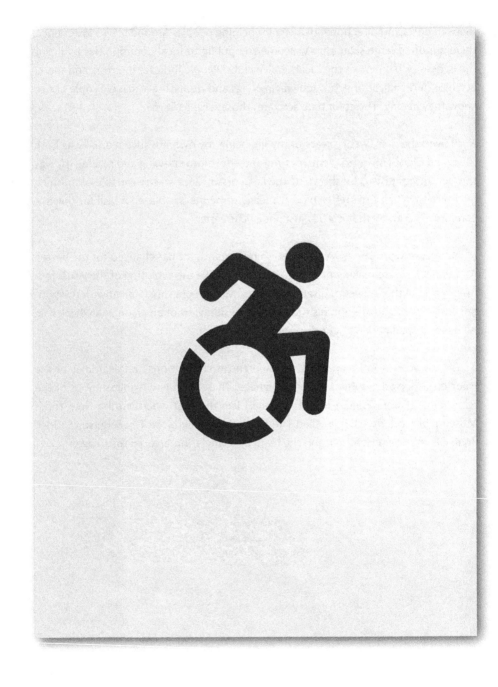

Their project intended to redesign the International Symbol of Access. The new version shows a person in forward motion, serving as a driver of their own life...rather than being in a passive position, ready to be pushed to a destination.

Since discovering theirs, I have seen these other two designs as well.

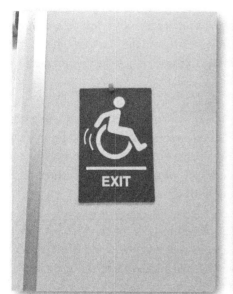 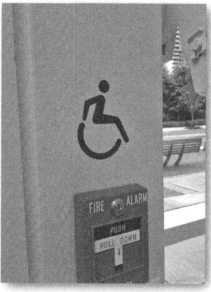

When I see the new images, I can relate to them far more than the traditional one. I internalize the new symbol's forward motion as a representation of me overcoming challenges and being the person I want to be and need to be.

There is only one blue sign that is a turn-off to me: the universal wheelchair logo and a red circle line through it. That signifies no available access to people who use wheelchairs. When I see it, I look at it as a cop-out. It comes off to me as the people in charge are telling me I can't go somewhere, instead of taking the time to find a way to make it accessible. I guess the ADA can change accessibility, but not people's attitudes.

Architects prefer to design parking lots with the handicapped parking stalls in the front of the main entrance of the building. This is a good idea, unless the building is older and with some kind of architectural or historical significance. As outlined in the ADA, if an accommodation is reasonable and feasible, it needs to be made. Under that interpretation, there are a lot of gray areas. For example, under the law, it is not reasonable or feasible to knock down fifty stairs and build a ramp to the front door of a historically famous landmark or building.

Often, the facility still needs to make some kind of accessible route to accommodate. They may design entrances that are placed into the back or side of the building. This may result in placing the location of the entrance the farthest distance away from where I'm given to park.

This situation forced me to invent the 3/2, 2/3 rule of accessibility. My rule states, "A person with a disability who must use an accommodation designed by an able-bodied person to overcome a physical barrier will have to travel three times as far and put in twice the effort. Or, they will have to travel twice as far and work three times harder than an able-bodied person to accomplish the same task."

In a perfect world, an accommodation would promote the shortest and easiest route for me to gain access to it. I have learned well that the world is not perfect. However, my understanding and belief in my rule makes all of the extra work I have to put in to accommodating my difference a little easier, both mentally and emotionally, because I'm already expecting it.

Accessible does not always mean inclusive. When I have to use the ramp and the person I'm with uses the stairs because it's easier for them, it separates us. Separate is not equal. Thankfully, engineers are finally acknowledging this when designing new environments, integrating a new approach to make things accessible for everyone.

Architects call it universal design. The concept was coined by the architect Ronald L. Mace to describe designing all products and the built environment to be aesthetically pleasing and usable to the greatest extent possible by everyone, regardless of their age, ability, or status in life.

I came across my favorite example of physical universal design when I was exploring the downtown riverfront area in Detroit, Michigan. I was in front of General Motors Renaissance Center and its five-story Wintergarden Atrium landing. The entrance of the building transitions to the International Riverfront through the use of a series of stairs shown here.

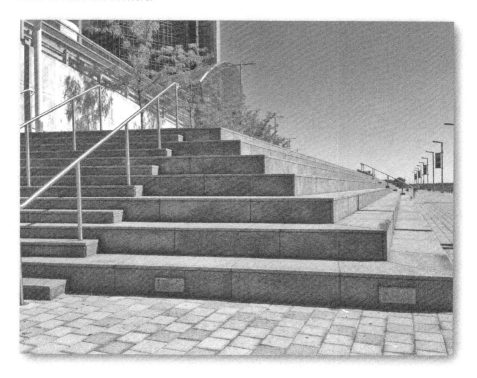

The first time I saw the space in real life, I was disheartened by the appearance of such a large and long series of steps. I thought the stairs were perfect to frame the space between the landing and the building. But once again, I would be denied traditional access to a public space due to the designer's preference to maintain a certain look.

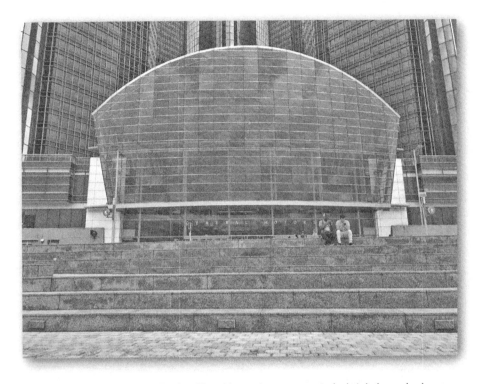

I pushed my chair hundreds of feet along the pavers nestled tightly to the bottom stairs. My eyes skimmed the lines of the steps, searching for the familiar break plane that signifies the entrance to a ramp. The parallel lines continued.

It wasn't until I reached the other end of the stairs that I noticed what had been so marvelously hidden: a fully ADA-compliant, accessible ramp, integrated so smoothly and perfectly that it proved to be invisible when viewed from the front of the board-walk. The design allowed me access to the facility, and it serves the larger purpose of integrating everyone into the same functional space. At the same time, this ramp met and exceeded the needs of people walking, riding their bikes, pushing strollers with young children, and those like myself with a wheelchair.

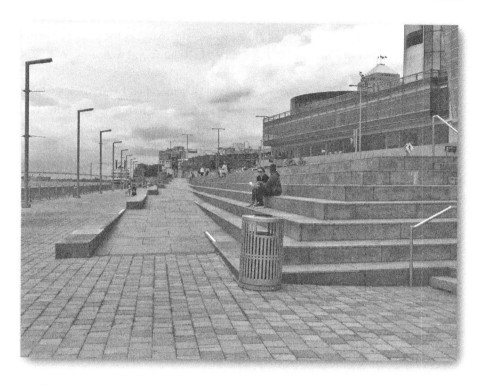

The space perfectly illustrates the spirit and intentions behind universal design by demonstrating equitable access and full utilization for everyone.

I look forward to the days in the future when universal design is the standard for all new construction. The idea of inclusion for people with disabilities isn't about changing the rules to accommodate; it's about including everyone and their abilities from the beginning.

Imagine what it would look like if everyone built their homes with the foresight to understand what their future situation might look like. Family members might eventually not be able to walk or climb stairs as easily as before. Their lives could be much easier if they already had doors that were wide enough to fit a wheelchair through for a future family member who might come to live with them.

On one of my last speaking tours, while I was staying at a hotel, I decided that I would like to go for a swim. It is a good form of exercise for me because I don't wear out my tires from using the treadmill. Just joking—the mats on the treadmill aren't wide enough for my wheels. Ever the rebel, I tried it. It didn't end well.

I love to swim. My act of swimming looks like a modified breaststroke, while I shake my butt like a mermaid. After swimming for forty-five minutes, I got out, dried myself off, and made my way back to my room. As I passed the front desk, the manager engaged me in conversation, saying, "We put in the handicapped pool lift for you, and you didn't even use it."

I responded, "Yes, I saw it and I'm really glad you have it. There are many people with mobility impairments that would need to use it. I'm just not one of those people."

I further explained, "I hadn't seen one like that before, and I did try to check it out. But when I pushed the buttons it wasn't working."

He acknowledged, "Yes, I know. We put it in to help, but we removed the batteries because people were using it like a diving board."

People are willing to make the investment into providing accommodations. Yet, I find that I have to bear the brunt of not using them, even when I don't need them. There are times, though, when in the presence of managers or owners of businesses, I will use one of their accommodations mainly to ease or assuage their feelings. I try to prevent them from becoming resentful of me for not using something that, in their minds, they put in just for me.

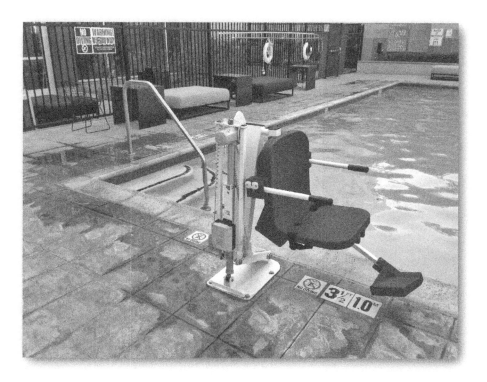

Most adaptations or modifications made to accommodate people are very well planned and implemented perfectly. However, a few mistakes are made from time to time.

The first mistake I see more often than anything else is a door on an accessible bathroom stall that opens inward toward the toilet. I can understand how an installer simply screws the door-swinging lock stop with the tab facing out just like all the other stalls in the bathroom. The problem with this is, as the door opens into the stall, it takes up the same space inside the stall that my wheelchair requires. This forces me to undress, transfer to the toilet seat, and do my business in full view of everyone walking past.

The second mistake I notice is when people install handicapped parking places incorrectly. The following photo is a good example of moderately well-placed accessible parking signage taken at a college where I was speaking. Unfortunately, there are a few problems with the installation, if you need to use the spaces.

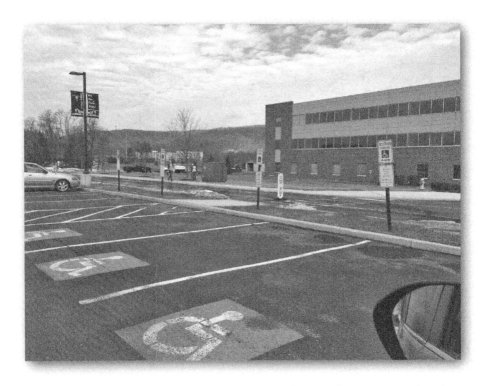

The width of each space is too narrow, given their configuration. Putting these spaces too close to each other is problematic. Without the additional required space for the no-parking cross-hatched accessible exiting area, there isn't a way for a person with a handicapped accessible van to get our wheelchairs out of the sides of our vehicles.

Additionally, there is the absence of curb cuts in and around these spaces. A person with a wheelchair needing to access the main entrance must first find a ramp or curb cut to access the sidewalk.

In order for me to get into the building, I had to follow the driveway out of the parking lot, cross into the intersection, and enter the cul-de-sac along with the moving vehicles. Some were even dropping off passengers—that's where the only curb cut was for the entire parking lot was. Oops!

I'm sure the parking lot planner for this Taco Bell wasn't really thinking of how anyone would use the ramp along with their parking space. How could the person and their wheelchair have access to the ramp...if the ramp was under their front bumper? Oops!

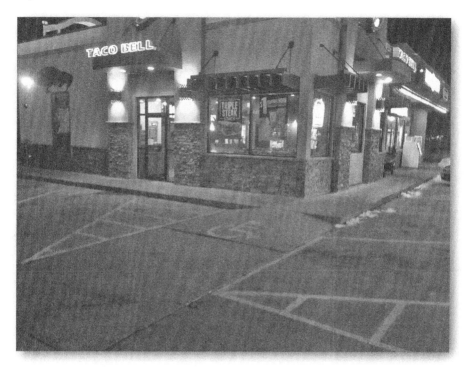

Thanks to the ADA and over twenty-five years of implementation, I can practically have the same expectation of physical accessibility that able-bodied people take for granted. Still, I find that people have certain expectations—low expectations—of me and my abilities. Oh, if they only knew!

POINT TO PONDER: Where do you think the ADA falls short? What could be improved?

The principles of universal design can help us evolve our thinking on the historical view and models of disability.

Traditionally, the idea of disability has been one of a "deficiency" or "abnormality." People with a disability are "afflicted" or "burdened" by it, and they seek a cure or treatment administered by a professional in hopes to become "normal." In many cases, a doctor would prescribe "treatment" or "arrangements" between the individual and society. The focus of any disability and responsibility for it, is all on the individual.

The broader approach of integrating the fundamentals of universal design leads to looking at disability through the lens of a broader social justice and civil rights model—one in which the burden of a disability is not placed on the individual, but instead on their society. The view is not that the person with disabilities is incomplete or not perfect to function in society; instead, it's that the environment they are forced to operate within highlights their challenges. A universally designed space offers a better opportunity to accommodate everyone while lessening the stigma of people who are regarded as being disabled.

This new view is based on the concepts of human rights and equality, including freedom from discrimination. Human variation is natural and vital in the development of dynamic communities. Disability is a social/political category that includes people with a variety of conditions who are bound together by common experiences (oppression and marginalization). Inclusion and full participation are a matter of social justice and civil rights. Disability is just another aspect of diversity.

PART 4

One Day at a Time

CHAPTER 1

Just Me

O ften, people come up to me and say how proud they are of me. "For what?" I want to ask—and sometimes I do. "For being out in public," they'll answer. "For getting out of bed," "For being capable," "For living your life."

These people say they view me as an inspiration—a concept I can't help but scoff at. Yes, they may view me as such, and if so, that's fine for them.

I understand that some people call me an inspiration because of the extra work it takes me to do the same things as other people. I find myself unworthy of that word. I do not view myself as an inspiration. I am not putting my life on the line in a battle zone, on a fire truck, or solving the world's problems. It just takes me a little longer to get off the sofa, carry my drink back to the coffee table, and sit back down.

To illustrate a person who is truly inspirational to me, I'd like to share with you a story about someone who, in my opinion, deserves the respect and honor bestowed on him.

I had the opportunity to educate a group of elementary school students in Wisconsin about the challenges of my everyday life. It was the second program of the day, and it ended as it usually does: with a well-fought wheelchair basketball game between a talented volunteer from the audience and myself. The cheering and applause rang out like thunder; I stood in front of the group and asked if I had delivered all of the fun I had promised, and they greeted my question with a resounding "Yes!"

I thought the teaching was done and I tried to catch my breath. Just at that moment, I was informed that there was one more story to be shared.

An adult member of the school took center stage to talk about a second-grade student in the audience named Levi. She told us all that it was a special day for Levi because he was in good health and spirits, and he had brought some very special items to share with the school.

Two years before, Levi was diagnosed with leukemia—specifically, acute lymphoblastic leukemia. Many of the students knew of him being in and out of school and were aware that Levi had many days when he didn't feel well, even while at school.

The teacher asked Levi to come to the front of the group with a few friends to help him share his story. Immediately, every hand in the gym went up. Everyone wanted to be with him. The pride on his face and the look in his eyes as he got to share the mo-ment with a lucky few were priceless. Two students were chosen to join Levi onstage. They were ready to do whatever they could to be with and to assist their friend.

The teacher brought out several large groupings of beads threaded on five neck-laces. Each necklace was well over twenty inches long and each one required its own second grader to hold it up and stretch it out on display. Levi and both members of his crew took responsibility for one of the necklaces. At the last moment, I came to the line of service because I saw that there were still two necklaces to be displayed.

We all held up Levi's art for everyone to appreciate. And then, we learned what each bead represented. Each individual bead was a symbol of courage that commem-orated milestones Levi had achieved along his unique treatment path.

The explanation of each individual bead was breathtaking. The small blue beads represented clinic visits. Each white bead was earned for completing a dose of che-mo. The red beads were for blood or platelet transfusions. We learned that a black bead represented the prick of a needle and saw that on each of Levi's necklaces there weren't just one or two black beads—there were twenty or more. The explanations of each bead went on and on, each decoration representing an act of courage and strength, greater than the last. The green beads were for lumbar punctures and spinal taps. All the magenta beads were for emergency room visits. Lime beads represented instances of neutropenia (low white blood cell count), fever, or a stay in isolation; light green beads were awarded for x-rays, CT scans, and other tests; yellow for a hospital stay; brown for hair loss. Levi was particularly proud of his glow-in-the-dark beads, which represented radiation treatments.

Everyone in the room could see exactly what Levi had already overcome. The weight of a fight against cancer was carried on the shoulders of this eight-year-old boy, and the proof of Levi's strength and courage was all there on 100 inches of thread.

Physically, I felt the weight of the beads in my arms. I had been holding only two strands up over my head for what seemed to be an eternity while being immersed in the story of how each bead was earned. As the teacher read, I could feel the burn in my shoulders, the weight of what I was holding. It was as if my arms could feel the weight of each individual bead as its description was read. My arms ached.

I, the over-forty-year-old Paralympic athlete and "role model" for this school, was credited with overcoming challenges and adversity. I was the one who was congratu-lated for enduring the pain of an offhand, insensitive comment from a stranger, or the challenge of carrying my wheelchair up a flight of stairs in an effort to enter a less than accessible building. The truth is: I have no idea if I could hold up even two-fifths of the representation of the weight of Levi's disease.

Nothing I have ever been through begins to compare to what Levi had already seen and experienced. His innocent eyes still held the sparkle of a child, his rosy red cheeks were full of love to give, and his smile showed that he knew joy and happiness. I only hope I can live up to his example of strength and perseverance.

Levi is true inspiration, genuine motivation, and a hero to myself and everyone else who has had the honor of meeting him. Levi is a boy who has already overcome struggles that would break a man.

It is amazing to think that he isn't out of the woods yet and still has many more beads to earn. But I assure you that Levi has an amazing, loving, and supportive family to help see him through. He's giving it the best he's got.

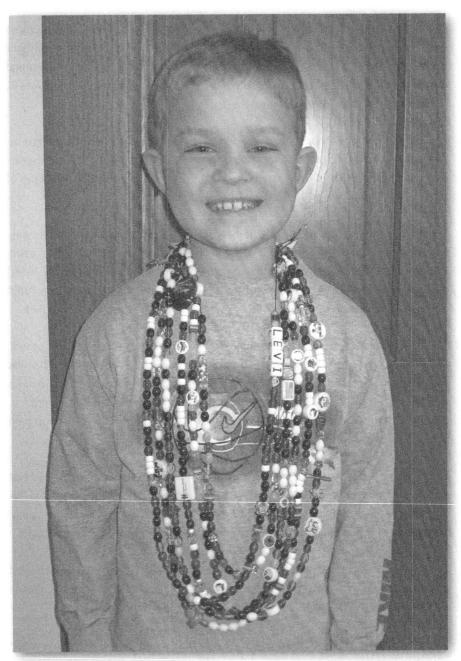

If you would like to learn more about the Beads of Courage program or to make a donation, visit www.beadsofcourage.org to read more of Levi's story

Most of my life, I have not felt that I was like Levi at all. He is worthy of being inspiring, but I am not. There is nothing phenomenal about how I get through a day. It's just what I do. I shower, I put clothes on, I have breakfast, and I just do my thing. I live my life, just as you live yours.

As I age, I find that I am losing the connection to the nobility that comes with being labeled as an inspiration. I have tried to assign additional intrinsic value to my struggles of attempting to accomplish the same tasks as able-bodied people. I try to believe it affords me extra credit toward being a better person. Now, though, all I see is everyone else's different challenges. I am left to find everyone I meet to be inspirational to me. I perceive my "issues" to be less than those of most other people's, and they walk.

CHAPTER 2

Independence

People always ask me if it is all right to hold the door open for a person who uses a wheelchair or offer help to someone who is disabled and might be in need of assistance. My response? I have a general rule I like to share: If you would do it for someone else, do it for me.

The easiest expression of this is to look at your own life. I call it the "good person test." Are you the person who would willingly hold the door open for another person behind you as you pass through a door? If you are, you qualify.

Most of the time, it is out of courtesy and/or respect for another person. If you have that respect for other people, have it for me and please hold the door for me.

I am just looking for the same treatment you would offer others. I am not expecting an extraordinary experience out of perceived guilt for another person's situation.

In the parking lot at Target, as I am heading toward the doors, someone who is 100 feet away might see and come running to help me with the door. Just as we meet at the door, the electric door slides open and we both feel a little silly.

Be aware of one other factor. I call it the angry disabled person syndrome.

You might know what I am talking about. It shows itself when you engage in a typical "helping" experience that you would have with anyone. But in this case, you are helping a person with a disability. Surprisingly, the person you are holding the door for looks at you and says with contempt and viciousness, "I can do that by myself."

I identify that as a symptom of the angry disabled person syndrome. Unfortunately, I have to admit, I was afflicted with it myself for many years. It resulted from the many times people tried to help me every day. There would come a point when I just wanted to be left alone and handle things by myself. When I reach that point, the anger monster within me rears its ugly head.

What I needed to do to overcome the syndrome was change my view. As I was letting the pressure of the over accommodation build within me, I had the wrong viewpoint. I was incorrectly internalizing the reason why people were helping me. I believed they thought I couldn't do anything by myself. I assumed that in their minds, they were judging me as an invalid. I believed that they thought, *It's lucky that I am here, because he probably can't do this by himself.*

It manifested itself into negative interactions with other people. On the good days, I would simply say with a bit of contempt, "Oh no, I got it." But on the bad days, I found myself barking back with some gruffness in my voice, "I can do it by myself!"

Finally, I decided I didn't like the person I was becoming. I saw myself driving people away because of my negative inner voice that was telling me they were doing it because they thought I was crippled, not that they were doing it as a nice thing because they hold the door for everyone else, too.

I didn't like how it was making me feel, so I did my best to try to put myself in the other person's shoes, to understand how they might have been feeling.

Most of the time, I have a high expectation for how good human nature can be. When people offer assistance to me, now I believe it is not because I use a wheelchair. It is offered because they are good people with only good intentions to help any per-son out of courtesy and respect.

It is quite admirable that people born and raised in the United States generally teach the value of having courtesy and respect for everyone, especially for those less fortunate than ourselves.

I find that the need for help looks different in the mind of the Millennial generation. In the past, members of a previous generation's words contributed to my perception of why people were offering help. It fed my negative inner voice. Out of the blue, for no apparent reason, strangers shopping around me would offer to reach something for me while saying, "Let me get that for you. You probably can't do it by yourself."

Today, when I am shopping and there is a Millennial around me, they don't say anything. If I do need help and ask them for it specifically, they say, "At first I saw you, and thought I should offer to help you. Then I realized that if you needed help, you would probably ask."

Perfect! This is an example of a generation changing their expectations of others. They expect people to be able to do things for themselves. I view it as progress toward a better understanding of other people's potential. They are seeing me as capable and not always in need of help.

This all leads back to Disability Privilege. Accommodations made from people offering assistance are the purest expressions of Disability Privilege. Very few people want to be the person who doesn't help out, as this is often considered socially unacceptable...or downright rude. Think about the able-bodied guy who's in a hurry and parks in the last handicapped spot. This can result in different reactions from others; perhaps a monetary fine for parking unlawfully or receiving a dirty look by passers-by. Our social upbringing gives us an understanding of the "right thing to do."

However, these reactions can flow in both directions.

I have learned that when a person doesn't have the information needed to handle a "helping out" situation, we, the receivers of the assistance, don't have the right to judge the quality of their character. We don't know their life experiences, and we should not judge the intention of their behavior.

When the host at a restaurant doesn't pull out a chair for me at a table at which I will be obviously seated, I could assume that they don't care about me personally, nor do they care about my experience with their establishment. I think, *This is not a good person because they are not doing their best to accommodate my needs. They should have done the right thing and pulled out the chair for me.*

I—or anyone else in the vicinity—may see this and pass judgment on the host because they aren't "doing the right thing," assuming that they have no compassion or don't care about accommodating me.

There are several things to consider, though. While many may consider the host's actions rude, I actually prefer to use the existing chair that is set at the table. I will transfer myself to it, and, if I am able, keep my wheelchair next to me. I'm able to manage on my own, and this is exactly what I'm hoping others will see. In fact, if the host wanted to include me with regard to seating, they could have mentioned, "I assume you can handle yourself, but please make me aware of any special accommodations you may require." That recognition also preserves my dignity with the assumption of my ability to handle myself.

If the host said those words, it would signify to me that an acknowledgement was made to the societal moral construct of helping people who might be worse off than another person.

I have always been fascinated by how or what people think is actually helpful. People hand me an umbrella when it rains. I know they are trying to help, but what they fail to understand is if I am holding an umbrella I can only push in circles. It also becomes a huge sail attached to my wheelchair, blowing me around in the storm. Their intentions are good, but the manifestation of their efforts does not prove to be helpful. Sometimes, their trying to help actually does more harm than good.

POINT TO PONDER: Have you ever found yourself trying to help, but actually doing the opposite?

Exiting from a recent airline flight, I waited for everyone to disembark the plane. Then, I made my way to the front. I found my wheelchair there and I transferred myself onto it.

I was traveling with two carry-on bags. Normally, my computer bag hangs off the back of my wheelchair, and my clothing bag hangs around my neck or off my shoulder. Both bags weigh a little over thirty-five pounds each. I positioned them as such and started making my way up the jet bridge.

Pilots, flight attendants, and service gate staff were quick to offer assistance. They wanted to help, but they also wanted to leave as soon as they could...as I did. I commented, "No thank you, I got it. I really can do it by myself."

I proceeded to make my usual joke: "I do this for a living."

I say that sometimes because actually, I do. I live my life, find ways to manage the accessibility challenges I face and share my observations as a professional presenter.

I hope my conversations with everyone I meet and get to talk to at movie theaters, post offices, and restaurants bring smiles and a new understanding. But on this particular day at the airport, I missed the mark.

I thought they had understood that I could manage the trip up the jet-way with no assistance. As I reached the second extension of the jet-way ramp, the ramp got sig-nificantly steeper for a short distance. I just couldn't push the wheel rims on my chair to move. I had to grab hold of a handrail on the wall for a moment to pull myself up toward the next, longer and less steep area of the ramp. I was able to do it of course, but it slowed me down and I had to shift my weight on the seat of my chair to accommodate the greater incline.

Just as I leaned forward into the railing, one of the co-pilots pushed on the highest point on the back of my wheelchair backrest and exclaimed, "Here you go, buddy!"

I do not have handles on the back of the wheelchair. When he pushed on the upholstery of my backrest, it immediately caused me to be thrust forward, and I fell off the front of my wheelchair.

The weight of my bag and its position on my chest prevented me from being able to stretch out my arms and catch myself. I had to let go of the handrail on the wall to try to catch myself. And when I did, with a horrendous thud, I came crashing down on the hard, cold, wet and dirty jet-way ramp. To make matters worse, my computer bag and all of my things dumped out in front of me as well.

As I was falling forward, the co-pilot jumped forward with me, falling over the back of my wheelchair, almost as if he was going to be able to grab my shoulders and pull me back upright. But he had no leverage. He had nothing to grab on to, and no way to actually give help. There was nothing to save either one of us from falling for-ward. I gasped, and he yelled, "Holy shit, I'm sorry" as he fell on top of me.

He rolled off of me sideways, apologized again, and said, "I know you said you could do it, but it looked like you still really needed help."

I did not get physically injured, but my ego was bruised. The last thing I ever want to do is fall out of my wheelchair, especially in front of people. I know it really makes me look disabled.

What bothered me the most, though, was that I had shared with the male co-pilot the idea that I was competent and capable not only of managing my way up the ramp, but also of taking care of myself.

The problem, in my mind, developed when he chose not to believe that I knew what was best for me in the situation, even after he asked. He could not believe me; he felt the need to offer assistance in the least productive manner possible, without even warning me. Ten minutes earlier, my life was in his hands on board the aircraft. Now, we both came crashing to the floor of the jet-way.

I understand that he might have seen part of his job to be one of a "protector." But protection can be compassionate or it can serve to ridicule a person if it doesn't reflect an accurate assumption of another person's capabilities. A good example of this could be when a man steps in to protect a woman without sizing up the situation and understanding if she has the situation well in hand.

It led me to believe that, in addition to not having legs, I also had no credibility to know when I might need assistance or when I could manage myself.

I am appreciative of the help, truly. But sometimes, in cases like these, it can back-fire. When someone is offering assistance of any kind, I say, "Thank you for the consideration, but I'm totally good."

If I think that what they are offering will help, I will accept. Either way, I measure their intentions and try to be appreciative.

POINT TO PONDER: Has anyone ever tried to help you when you were fully capable of handling whatever the situation was? How did it make you feel?

CHAPTER 3

The Platinum Rule

f I had to list one aspect of being disabled that still shocks me, it is that huge numbers of people still treat me as "less than" able-bodied people. Sure, my lack of legs might cause me to take longer to do certain tasks, but that doesn't make me less successful, less aware, or less human than the next guy.

Dr. Tony Alessandra developed an alternative to the Golden Rule, which might be more appropriate when bridging cultural differences. He named it the Platinum Rule: "Treat others the way they want to be treated." The message in this chapter can be boiled down to my version of that: "Treat me normally, like everyone else."

I found myself shopping at Whole Foods in Madison, Wisconsin a few weeks ago. It is not my first grocery store of choice, but I appreciate their fresh ground almond butter and their house brand of unsweetened iced tea.

Behind three other customers, I was in the checkout line with all of my items. I'm not sure how you feel about people who ask you for donation money in front of others, but I really don't like it. No, not because I don't want to give, but because I feel it places unwarranted pressure on me to give. I also think that people make judgments about me based on whether or not I give anything.

As I was waiting in line, looking at the latest cover of *People* magazine, I overheard the checkout person making a plea to one of the customers ahead of me. Waiting until the transaction was almost complete, the checker asked the customer, "Would you like to contribute a dollar to the needy?"

My immediate thought was, *Oh great, looks like I am going to be guilted into giving a dollar now.*

Keep in mind, to me, it is really *not* about the money. I can afford the dollar. It's just the circumstance in which they ask that bothers me.

Then, I heard the customer reply, "No."

I was happy because I felt like someone else might feel like I did about the intrusion. As the next customer's items were being scanned, she was presented with the same question. "Would you like to donate a dollar to the needy?"

"No, thank you."

She had declined as well. *This is great,* I thought. I could feel the anxiety slowly leave my body because now I knew the answer I was going to give the checker.

It was finally time for the third person in line to check out. She was a younger woman between twenty-five and thirty. "Would you like to donate a dollar to the needy?" the checker asked.

She replied, "Sure."

That was when things changed for me. He stopped what he was doing and raised his eyes from the register. His face lit up and he looked directly at her, saying, "I just want you to know that I really appreciate you donating this money. The cause is local and really great, and I can tell you are a wonderful person."

Wow, was I blown away. Not only did I change my mind about giving a dollar, but for that kind of validation, I was now looking forward to it!

I smiled in anticipation as I watched my items advance on the automated belt. I met the gentleman's eyes and raised my eyebrows in a meaningful and engaging way... Then, I proceeded to pay for my groceries. Wait! He didn't even ask me if I would like to give to "needy" people.

I stayed in the moment long enough for it to be a bit awkward, but then I spoke up, "I'd like to donate a dollar!"

He was surprised for an instant, then nonchalantly said, "Okay." He had a small look of surprise on his face as I presented a single dollar bill from my wallet and went on my way. This was not exactly the situational response I was hoping for, but at least I helped by donating.

I will never know what he was thinking that day. Maybe he had met his donation quota for the shift. Or, perhaps much like other people, he thought I was part of the "needy" class because I don't have legs. I like to think he just realized I was overpaying for my gourmet peanut butter, and he didn't want to ding me again.

I probably could have worked a little harder in the moment to wait and see if he would ask. It might have allowed me to take a proactive role in the conversation and possibly break down a stereotype he could have been buying into. Sometimes, though, I don't want to wave my educational flag. I just want to pay for my groceries and be on my way.

Later that week, I was shopping by myself at an outdoor mall when I noticed an older woman struggling with holding the door open for herself and managing all of her packages. I thought I could assist by holding the door for her.

I like to play with "walkies." I call people who walk "walkies" for fun. In almost every situation, people hold the door for me as I roll through. I like to run ahead and hold the door for able-bodied people.

I briskly walked over to her, grabbed hold of the door, and held it for her as she walked through. I looked at her briefly enough to notice that all she did was look down at where she thought my legs should have been.

I understand the nature of difference. When we, as humans, see something for the first time that is out of the ordinary, we stare at it for a brief time to comprehend what we are seeing and develop some understanding of the situation.

If I were in class and someone invited a pink elephant into the room, I would have to pay attention to the elephant. I might even have a few questions for the elephant. I would not think it was impolite to consider the nature of its difference. When people see me for the first time, I allocate a certain amount of time for them to comprehend the absence of my legs. Then, I try to direct their attention to my face and eyes. Upon my eyes greeting theirs, I extend a wink and a greeting to let them know that I am friendly and courteous.

For me the challenges surrounding the next part of the interaction have everything to do with their age and how they were raised to interact with someone they perceive as disadvantaged or different compared to themselves. The correct societal teaching on how to interact with a person who has a disability has changed over the years.

I still remember being taught when I was young that it was impolite to stare at someone less fortunate than myself. When I interact with people my age and older, if they choose to look at me at all, many times it is with "poor, poor, pitiful you" eyes. Some will actually shield their eyes with their hands.

There are people I will never meet because they see me first and quickly turn the corner to avoid interacting with me. Some people hide. I will never know about the ones who are really good at it. Their actions are the opposite of tolerance—it's intolerance by omission. But when avoiding looking at or interacting with someone different from you, who is that really "protecting"? Am I avoiding the situation to protect myself? If I perceive theirs is a worse life than mine, by not observing it, am I protecting myself from feeling that I need to offer some kind of help? Is this a root cause of Disability Privilege?

For the most part, generations younger than mine have been educated by priori-tizing diversity, inclusion, and the positive aspects of curiosity. Individuals like these are more likely to interact with me in a casual way, sparking conversations with a ques-tion or just smiling at me as we pass.

When I am exposed to the behavior and energy of an older person (one who was educated like I was), it sucks the pleasant disposition right out of me. I feel like I'm forced into a defensive posture. Not having the ability to effectively demonstrate values associated with how "normal" I could be in fewer than ten seconds leaves me feeling unsettled.

As for the older woman for whom I was holding the door, I did not have a chance to meet her eyes because she was completely fascinated with the absence of my legs. It was a bit off-putting in the way I assume it would be for a woman who was trying to have a conversation with a man who would rather look at certain body parts than her eyes.

The real shame came upon me when, without a look to address my eyes or any kind of acknowledgement of me as a person, she blurted loudly, "I did *not* need to see that today!"

She was referring, of course, to my situation—the absence of my legs and how that negatively impacted her day.

I do claim to be fast on my feet with comments for everyone—I always have something to say. But when she struck me with that verbal jab, I was dumbstruck. Never before have I had someone treat my basic existence with such disdain. Just by her witnessing my situation, I somehow contributed to ruining her day. Her words were like a kick to my chest that knocked the wind out of me.

It hurt really bad—so much so, I drove the two-and-a-half-hour trip back to my home in Wisconsin with tears in my eyes. How could I have such a terrible effect on a stranger? When I arrived home, I shared the moment with my wife. She explained something to me that I wished I had figured out myself.

I gave all that time in the car to being hurt and upset by a person whom I will probably never see again, a person who played no role forming the man I was or will ever be, a person who holds no power of influence over anything I value. I made the mistake of caring what she thought and said.

I should have realized that she was just an "angry and miserable able-bodied person."

Lifelong experiences helped me frame what I learned from the woman at the mall that day. Someone who becomes an "angry...person" has a greater disability than a disabled person with a positive outlook.

When people say things to me, I have to believe that what they are saying is, at a minimum, partially true. When I want to react badly to their words, I need to remember that the part of me that is hurting is reacting to the truth I have disconnected from in order to protect the bigger better person, I want to be.

Some people try to keep others from speaking the truth by saying things like "You can't say things like that to people because it's not nice."

By using those words, aren't we really trying to protect other people from themselves when we say phrases like "That may be true, but don't tell them that. It will hurt their feelings because they don't want you to perceive that of them" or "They don't want to admit that to themselves."

The woman for whom I held the door might be frightened of aging. Seeing me may have reminded her of her own discomforts. She could be internalizing her possible future use of a wheelchair because of a progressively degenerative disease.

Her interaction with me and on that day could have been the first moment she was forced to confront her reality. Maybe up to that point, she had just seen her granddaughter kick her first soccer goal. She could have just completed her first watercolor painting in a class she was taking. Or her current condition had slipped her mind because the warmth of the mid-afternoon breeze took her back to a vacation she went on with her late husband.

I could have legitimately ruined her day by figuratively slapping her in the face with the reality of my existence. I blanched at her words when she claimed to "not need to see 'that' today." I internalized her words as a slight when in truth, she could have just been telling me something more pressing and painful in her world.

Very few people share their truth with me without at least trying to form it in a way to protect my feelings. Maybe her crassness could teach me more about myself.

The most difficult times for me are when I perceive the existence of my disability as having a negative impact on others. When that occurs, I just find myself saying "I'm sorry" a lot. Truthfully, though, I have nothing to apologize for...and I know that; however...

I was flying out of the Chicago Midway Airport, 6:00 AM flight, which required a 4:30 AM airport arrival. To save a little money, I parked in the economy parking garage.

I was not worried at all about taking the airport shuttle bus to the main terminal, because finally, twenty-five or so years since the ADA was passed, all of the airport's buses have wheelchair lifts. It's pretty standard nowadays.

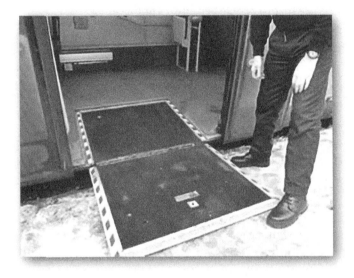

I was the only person getting on the bus at 4:30 AM. From the front seat, the driver, a middle-aged man, let out the pressure from the front- and side-wheel airbags. His actions lowered the overall height of the bus to accommodate the ramp and make it easier for me to use. He proceeded to walk to the side door and push a button that was supposed to unfold the ramp. The motors made a grinding noise, but the ramp didn't move.

Immediately, the driver looked at me and apologized. He told me this was his bus and yesterday, after his shift, he reported the ramp failure to the maintenance department. He thought it was fixed, but he didn't have a chance to check it yet, since this was his first ride of the day.

He told me not to worry and then said, "I got this."

He reached into his pocket and produced what looked like a butter knife. He wedged it in between the floor and the ramp and levered the ramp up just enough for the action of the motor to fully extend the ramp.

Needless to say, I was impressed. I was on my way without a second thought.

The following morning, though, was a little different. I landed back at Midway around 10:00 AM. It was snowing so much that we were notified that ours was the last plane allowed to land before an all-stop was issued for the entire airport. Man, did I feel lucky! It may have been a short trip, but there is still no place like home.

I deplaned with the rest of the passengers and we all made our way to the ground transportation. Midway's outside drop-off point is under a series of cantilevered roofs that are offset just enough to allow rain or snow to still reach you if the wind is blowing. And it always is because, after all, Chicago isn't called the Windy City for nothing.

A large group of us was waiting for the economy parking bus while tensions were running high. Everyone was becoming agitated as we waited in the blistering cold wind and snow for the shuttle to come.

I was the first one to see the bus as it crested the turn, so I made my move. It's important for me to let the bus driver know that I am intending to board the bus with other people and alert him to the needs of my wheelchair. Those needs translate into the specific action of the driver to park close enough to the curb to allow for space for the ramp, all the while paying enough attention to allow the ramp to unfold equidistant between the four-foot-tall, eight-foot-long cement barriers.

Though I had established my presence in front of the crowd, I waved to the driver. He didn't acknowledge me and proceeded to find his perfect spot to stop. He drove the bus past where I was waiting, finally stopping, now leaving me at the rear of the bus. All of the other passengers pushed their way into the warm protection of the bus. I was left out on the curb.

I moved up the sidewalk and approached the driver at the front door; he was still in his seat after everyone loaded, paying attention to his phone hidden between his legs.

In an outdoor, strong voice, I asked him if he would pull forward to a better spot for me to board. He gave me a pursed look and waved me off to the side so he could pull up a bit closer.

The bus was now almost full, and everyone was ready to go. My boarding the bus was almost a cruel joke to play on all the impatient travelers.

After the bus crept forward and all the doors opened again, the other passengers on board shrank into their seats with the new blast of frigid air. By the looks on their faces and the physical gestures of moving closer to one another, I could tell that the people closest to the aisle were gauging where I was going to sit. All the seats were taken, and the luggage space was occupied with golf bags. I knew there was room for me at the edge of the ramp inside the bus. I could hold on, if I could just get in.

The ADA legislation does its best to guarantee equal access to people's buildings, but it doesn't do anything to guarantee access to people's patience.

Then, I remembered the small ramp snafu from the day before. I thought, *What are the chances of this bus being the same one?e?e?* I figured they must have at least fifteen different buses in the motor pool working different parts of the airport.

Sure enough, after the bus lowered, the driver walked back to use the switch to un-fold the ramp, and nothing happened. All of the passengers were watching the circus and didn't know what to do. I waited for the butter knife move, and it didn't happen. I was experiencing a new person, the same bus, and a completely different level of service.

I rolled closer to the driver; he looked at me and said to my astonishment, "How's this supposed to work?"

Was it my responsibility to know, and to tell him how to do his job? No—but in this case, at least I kind of did. I explained that if he had something to wedge into the edge, he could release the ramp like I saw the day before.

He looked at me in relative confusion. But then it was like a light went on in his head. He went back to the front of the bus and proceeded to take apart the plastic pieces under the front window. Behind the first aid kit, he grabbed some kind of tool and started back toward where I was still waiting.

When I looked through the windows of the bus, I could see men grimacing and looking at their watches. Others were making frustrated eye contact with strangers who, up until that time, had some compassion for my situation. Now, though, because all of the doors were still open on the bus, they were really cold—cold enough to flush the compassion right out of them.

I tried to express some compassion to those people who were sitting near the open doors. I distributed a series of quiet apologies. "Please forgive me. I know it is taking too much time, but I really need to get on this bus, too." I found a few empathetic glances.

One woman asked, "How could this be broken?"

A man wearing a veteran's Navy cap said, "The buses are always broken."

A little girl loudly exclaimed, "Mommy, I'm cold!"

The reality was that everyone was freezing, no one wanted to be there, and everyone was tired. Three strikes.

Moments later, the driver came back with the perfect tool, specifically made to wedge under the ramp to release it...but to no avail. There was no way for me to reach the driver to instruct or even help, so a very angry and somewhat deranged father leapt from his seat. He had previously been tending to his family's needs while witnessing our challenge. With his bare fingernails, he cleared out a portion of winter sludge from where the seam of the ramp met the floor. It was pure, brute strength that allowed his fingers to form the wedge and lift the ramp.

I met his eyes and gave him a heartfelt, visual, non-spoken thank you. He acknowledged it and moved back to his seat and his family.

I boarded the bus and grabbed a metal bar for stability. The rules for riding the bus while using a wheelchair state that all wheelchairs have to be strapped and locked down to the floor to keep the person using the wheelchair and the other riders on the bus safe.

I never want them to strap me down because I've had previous wheelchairs bent and broken due to the bus driver tying onto the wrong parts of my chair. I am always looking either for understanding from the drivers about my situation, or I bank on their incompetence in follow procedures. This driver didn't let me down when he walked right back to the driver's seat.

Confused, I looked around because I wanted to see if any other passengers had noticed that the ramp still fully deployed, doors open, and the airlift still down. The driver was about to pull away from the curb. The result could have been a nightmare.

Seeing the general look of concern from my fellow travelers, I now knew that it was my job to do something, and quickly. I grabbed the ramp switch and pushed up on the button. The ramp responded and came on board, but the doors were still open. At the same time that I activated the switch, other riders started yelling at the driver that the bus wasn't secure. People standing around me looked toward the front of the bus and yelled, "Stop!" "Wait!" "The doors aren't closed."

The driver, not aware enough to listen to anyone onboard, proceeded to shift the bus into drive. The action caused the horn to turn into a full alert notification system. The noise inside the bus was deafening. Children pushed their fingers inside their ears. People loudly gasped out of frustration. All eyes directed back at me again and people shook their heads, disgusted and frustrated.

I couldn't take the tension; I closed my eyes tightly and hung my head. I clung to the side of the bus where I had wedged myself as close to the folded ramp as I safely could.

The driver leapt out the front door of the bus, ran to the side door, jumped on the ramp three times for good measure, and, using all of his force, man-handled the doors to get them to close. He returned to the driver's seat and inflated the shock-absorbing airbags.

We were finally and safely on our way. My relief was momentary. Since I was the last one on, I would probably be the first one off.

I was only halfway through this bad dream. I had no idea how getting off the bus was going to work. I sat there and shook my head in sad surrender.

As soon as the bus came to a stop, I found myself apologizing again to everyone around me as they left. "I'm sorry. Really, I am sorry."

The super-fingered father pushed past me as I pressed my chair and myself into the crowd. He grabbed the edge of the ramp again and lifted it up, even before the bus lowered. He stood guard and let all the passengers in the back of the bus off and proceeded to guide me off the ramp. The people at the front of the bus evacuated through the front door.

I don't really know what happened with the bus or the driver as I left via the park-ing garage that day. However, I can assure you I could still hear the bus's horn blare as I made my way to my car.

I know that I shouldn't have to tell people that I am sorry and take unnecessary responsibility for broken public accommodations. The reason why I feel like I have to apologize is because I am still the one other people have to make sacrifices for because I'm "not normal." They wouldn't have had these problems if I wasn't there. The only reason why I can be there is because I survive on the goodwill and the best of intentions of others.

Just because I'm disabled and need extra assistance doesn't mean those people should take out their frustrations on me. I was just the unlucky one to be there in that moment. It could have been anyone in my situation.

POINT TO PONDER: Have you ever been blamed for something that was out of your control because of someone else's incompetence?

The ADA has given me the opportunity to live a life as normal as possible and be able to access much more of the world than ever before.

Rather than getting mad at me, perhaps it would be better if people directed their energy at asking why the ADA laws and accommodations aren't being maintained, such as the ramp on the bus. I'm fairly certain that the bus I was on is not the only one with maintenance issues.

What occurred on the bus was just a small example of a larger existing problem in terms of training, maintenance, and levels of service as part of an organization. Unfortunately, many of the timid take the easy way out, saying, "It is what it is," and then they dismiss it as an isolated instance of inconvenience.

When people with disabilities are denied service or access to something because an accommodation is broken or unusable, as an official member of a "protected class" in America, it can be defined legally as discrimination. Unfortunately, what everyone on the bus experienced was the secondary impact of discrimination toward a person who needs a reasonable accommodation to have equal access to travel. The ADA is making things better for disabled people, but I still see problems like these in our society.

POINT TO PONDER: Have you ever experienced a secondary impact from someone who is being discriminated against?

Sometimes, it's not people's actions toward me, but rather their words that hurt. How often on the news do I hear yet another story about the "crippling" impact of a weather event, be it a blizzard, a flood, or a tornado. I know they are not talking about me. But anytime I hear the word "cripple" used, my shoulders scrunch up a little bit, my face grimaces, and I shake my head.

Obviously, I am triggered by the word "cripple" being used several times a week to describe the damaging effects of something. "The people are experiencing the crippling effects of the hurricane." "The ship was crippled at sea when its engines failed." "The cripple was crippled by his crippling disease." Okay, I've never heard the last one on television, but it is interesting to see the word used as a noun, verb, and adjective in one sentence.

Intentions of newscasters are not to try to illustrate or promote a perceived inability or disability within a minority group. I believe the word holds negative connotations and is loaded with stigma. I view the word "cripple" as being outdated and inappropriate, much like the word "retarded." When people use it casually in all of its forms, I wish they could learn from the current, cultural disability nomenclature.

I know that the physical and emotional reaction I have is mine. I am internalizing their words based on how I want to see myself and how I wish to be seen by others. I wish they would have the self-awareness to know they are contributing to negative stereotyping of people with disabilities. But I am not going to throw a hammer through my television or burn down their building just because they are using a word which promotes labeling language.

When people use the word "crippled," I try to tell myself I am in the very small minority of people who get triggered by that word. I try not to get upset. The word does not revolve around me and my sensitivities...or my way of thinking. I have to measure their best intentions and realize that they're not purposefully trying to target me with that specific word. I find it better to remove myself from the situation or simply turn the channel.

It would be great if I wasn't a tourist in the able-bodied world. I know the best way for me to change the usage of the word is to have the conversation with people close to me. I ask them not to use it because I believe it promotes a negative view of people with a disability in general. I find that my friends are far less likely to use the word after we talk about it. I know I am far more likely to change the words I use if I know they negatively affect someone in my life, too.

POINT TO PONDER: What are the words or situations that trigger you? How do you handle it?

Unfortunately, a low expectations for people who are different are ingrained deep within our society, even in the ways we use our language.

Look at the words our society continues to use to define and describe a person with a disability. Most of them are nouns and adjectives that promote a less than adequate situation or expectation. Words that discriminate include: invalid, handicapped, disabled, crippled, gimpy, damaged, retarded, paralyzed, debilitated, and impaired. I am going to stop there, or I might hurt my own feelings. What is important here is the common characteristic of "deficiency" in all these words.

How can we not think of someone as being "less than" when the words we use to describe that person all have that connotation? Words mean things. They are our primary method of conveying our thoughts and ideas to others.

When people ask me what I want to be called, I tell them, "My name is Matt."

Unfortunately, that's not the answer they are looking for. Then they'll say, "Sure, but what are we supposed to call you people?"

I realize they are trying to politely ask what is the politically correct nomenclature I would like them to use to describe the larger group with which I identify. I proceed to explain that currently, the phrase "a person with disabilities" is considered to be best. It is im-portant to put the person first, but still acknowledge the context of their experience. They are a person first and always.

But I do go back to the beginning and say, "I really do prefer to specifically be called Matt." When meeting people and making friends, engage first in the traditional exchange of names and courtesies, while focusing on your commonalities. Then let each person's uniqueness reveal itself through the friendship over time. When you learn about the people before their disability, you can better serve as an advocate for them because you know who they are as a person, not as a disability stereotype.

My disability is a part of my experience, but it isn't all-encompassing. I have many interests and memberships in lots of groups and all of those combine to make me who I am.

POINT TO PONDER: If you could choose how strangers identified you, what are the words that you hope they would use?

One of the activities in which I participated was the local 5K fun run/walk called the Color Run. The energy at the event was magnetizing. With the music, dancing, and people, it was a great time, even if it took me a few days to wash out all the colorful dust thrown at me. My wheelchair also needed a good cleaning.

My first Color Run was also the first time I had done something like that, and with the new activity came lots of new people to meet. Strangers kept coming up to me and using words like "handi-capable" and "differently-abled" to describe my situation and participa-tion. One person said, "It looks like you have a disability, but it doesn't have you."

I wanted to appreciate the sentiment, but to me it came off as going too far, es-pecially when you consider that most of the people saying these things and inventing these new phrases are able-bodied. I feel like they are making up words to try to soften the impact of our disability on us *and on them*. If in their mind, they can put a posi-tive spin on my situation, my disability is easier for them to understand and deal with.

My favorite response I hear often is "It's great you're here, overcoming your disability!"

I always thank them because I know they mean it as a compliment. I can't blame them—I think that society has taught people that being disabled means to be inferior. When people choose to compliment me, I wish it would be more inclusive and they would speak to me as if we were both there as equals. They could connect with me by saying, "It was a great day for this event. It looks like we both had a ton of fun."

Even more concise and casual is, "Pretty awesome, right?"

I don't want them to compliment my ordinary actions as if they were extraordinary.

I try to put the "overcoming" comment in a different, diverse context to better understand it. Should people ever celebrate an African American's ability to overcome their challenges of being black? It sounds to me like saying, "Look how inspirational they are. It's almost like they're white."

My mind then jumps to how it is also incorrect to mention to an African American that you don't see their skin color.

A teacher at a diversity conference I attended explained the reason it is considered inappropriate to claim to be colorblind when referring to another person's outward appearance is primarily twofold.

The existence of white privilege in our society poses additional challenges to anyone who is not a Christian, heterosexual, white, land-owning male. Our forefathers established our country's societal norms and values when they created this union. Anyone who is not benefited by these privileges may have a harder time achieving success in this country because of the advantages shared with that majority class.

When a person tries to pay a compliment to anyone living in the United States who isn't white by saying they don't see their skin color, that individual fails to deliver their intended compliment. This is primarily because they are not acknowledging all the extra effort the member of the minority invests to accomplish the same thing as a white person.

Secondly, recognizing and celebrating "sameness" by not observing skin color promotes the idea that a person who is regarded as an "other" can only be valid as long as they can be recognized and celebrated for how well they fit into the perceived box of acceptability the member of the majority culture puts them into.

I continued to draw a parallel from that argument to all the times people approached me and said, "I don't even see your wheelchair. You are so able-bodied!"

I welcome a language that is inviting and not imposing, and in the past I had always taken that as a compliment. And after people say that to me, I actually have said out loud, "Winning!"

I don't know if it is appropriate for me to validate myself by how well able-bodied people tell me I am doing at making them not see my wheelchair. I have never really wanted people to tell me that they notice how much harder it is for me to bring in the groceries, paint a wall over five feet high, or put a kayak on the top of my truck. When they point those things out to me, I just hear them telling me I'm disabled and I'm different.

Every day, I recognize that the absence of my legs changes the way I do things. I was raised to see the benefits of fitting in without receiving extra credit or attention. My whole life I've simply been trying to be something I can never be: accepted by people I wish I was more like.

You might call it "overcoming." I call it "doing what I need to do to pass."

POINT TO PONDER: What kind of things do you do to be successful and pass as something you are not? How much effort are you willing to put into that process and why?

CHAPTER 4

A Place in Both Worlds

feel as if I have a place in both the able-bodied and disabled world.

While attending a positive psychology conference, I found myself at the back of the large convention hall looking for a glass of water. I had seen a gentleman enter the room after me, using an electric wheelchair as a mobility device. He had a "sip and puff" controller in his mouth. Many people can operate all the functions of their wheelchair through blowing or sucking on a straw connected to their chair's control box. Technology is truly amazing.

Over the natural progression of us finding our seats in the room, we both found ourselves gravitating toward the beverage table. I was a bit ahead of him in line, and, feeling like I could help someone else possibly in need, I offered to get him a steaming cup of coffee. He said that would be fine. I prepared the cup for him and placed it next to his hand on his armrest.

I tried to maintain eye contact with him and not stare at his chair or his condition. I didn't notice that his level of paralyzation rendered his hands and arms immobile and prevented him from taking the coffee from my grasp. As I released the cup, I assumed he would take it from me.

Nope.

I spilled lava-hot coffee on his hand and all over his chair. After a few minutes of cleanup with napkins, the chair and his clothing were fine. For me in the moment, I was glad and oddly relieved he couldn't feel the burns on his hand and arm.

I am ashamed to admit, when I see a person using a wheelchair out in public, I have what I believe to be a very able-bodied reaction. I wonder how and why they are there. Where did they park? What kind of a job could that person actually have because of their condition?

Then, I realize that this is probably what able-bodied people think of me. In that moment, I realize that I'm viewing the "lesser-abled" man in the wheelchair as many able-bodied people probably view me.

My identity exists both in the world of disability and in the world of the able-bodied. There have been many times when I have felt the urge to just start helping with-out taking the time to ask how to help. Or I feel the need to be nicer to people because I worry that they might not feel included. Disability Privilege is at work inside me as well. If it is very confusing for you, the reader, you can imagine the internal dialogue I have with myself daily because of all the years of conditioning I have gone through.

As I look back, I now realize that denial has served as a great coping mechanism for me. Ignorance, even if it is about our own condition, can be bliss. Even though denial may be a source of comfort for some, it can also become a crown of thorns, es-pecially when it comes to coping with reality. My denial over being disabled has been a double-edged sword because it has not always been negative.

POINT TO PONDER: Do you deny any aspect of your own life that may be hurting your overall growth?

I have experienced many positive things because I have never thought of myself as being disabled. There is a delicate balance in there somewhere. If I saw myself as disabled, then I might act the part. It's easy to do because of Disability Privilege. It gives and it takes.

I get treated quite well because of accessibility concerns and it really is nice to have doors opened for me. At the same time, it's annoying because this might mean I am viewed as "lesser than" and, therefore, deserving of pity.

Over the course of my life as I've tried to deal with challenges that most people experience, I have always rejected the idea of speaking to a therapist. I figured they wouldn't be able to help me with my real problems. I thought all they would want to do is talk about the fact that I don't have legs and how that challenge impacts my outlook and relationships.

Through my involvement in disabled sports, I have been fortunate enough to find a number of friends I can talk to about unique challenges I face. Not a lot of people know how challenging it can be to feel the head of a tack in my wheelchair tire, knowing that in the next five minutes the tube will either explode or fully deflate, and I will have to change it or push around on the rim of the wheel and try not to destroy it before I can get to a bike shop.

Once when I was at the grocery store, looking at the large variety and different colors of eggs, I asked the able-bodied woman standing next to me if she thought brown eggs tasted better than white eggs. She replied, "Oh, do you need me to reach some for you?" Uh, no. I was just asking about taste preferences—but thanks for the offer.

I find comfort in complaining to a wheelchair-using friend about people who can only think of interaction with me as a possible opportunity to "help."

My suspicions are usually confirmed about the professionals because every time I went to the doctor's office, they wanted to know everything about my disability. It even happens present day, and even if I am there with another person and I don't have the appointment. I end up having to explain to the medical staff that I was born without legs, there was no known cause, and that it has *nothing* to do with why my friend might have strep throat or why she skinned her knee playing softball. I am not today's patient.

My experience with doctors is that they always want to make it about the legs.

If I went to therapy, I feel like I would have to hold a sign that reads, *I don't want to be this thing that I am, so please don't bring it up. I don't want to have to react again to the reality that I don't fit into what is perceived and accepted as normal. Please don't be mean by being truthful. Don't make me confront what I am.*

I sometimes just want to scream out loud, in a large packed public place, "IT'S NOT ABOUT THE LEGS!"

The time I spend with my able-bodied friends really shows me how great being non-disabled is. It looks almost effortless for them to carry things, reach high places, and interact with each other on a physically higher plane. But, I do really enjoy my parking privileges.

Over the years, when I've taken time to reflect, I have wondered: *How much emotional stock and self-esteem have I invested in how well I can compete in the able-bodied world?*

I wonder if I should take pride in not having to use accommodations such as electric door openers or specialized lift van services designed by people who are trying to make my life better. On the flipside, I wonder if I am being selfish by not appreciating all of the advancements people have made for me and for those in somewhat similar situations. Since there is a stigma that comes with disability, I'll admit that I hide my handicapped parking authorization card when I'm not driving. I don't want people to see it and judge my driving and myself as defective.

Believe it or not, sometimes when I pull into the handicapped parking space, some people will actually stop and tell me I can't park there because they seem to think I look too able-bodied to qualify. When I open the rear door and show them the wheelchair, they apologize. For just a moment, it makes me feel victorious, like I won a little because I fooled them into thinking I was not disabled. I guess the only person I am truly fooling is myself.

I ask myself if I'm putting on an "able-bodied show" to try to accumulate points by playing some non-existent game mostly to win acceptance in the able-bodied world.

Do I just want to prove to them that I can do everything they can do? And, if I earn enough "able-bodied points," could I be normal like them or at least have the ability to truly pass as one of them?

POINT TO PONDER: Have you experienced wanting to be someone other than who you are, specifically because of a difference? Why is it so hard to simply accept who we are? Why are we competing?

I think back to when I was first going to school and the well-meaning adults who tried to push me into using prosthetic legs at an early age. I wonder now if I should have believed them when they said how much better my life would have been if I had learned to walk.

Whether I was walking around or not, I learned that the more I could "get over" other people's perceptions, the more opportunities I would have to be successful in the able-bodied world. It was the only world that mattered to me.

So, do I want legs?

After thinking about it, you bet your legs I do!

A few years ago, I was watching a documentary about children who experienced lifelong profound hearing loss. After exploring all the advances in cochlear implant technology, a number of kids decided to get the surgery that would give them the ability to hear.

The most impactful part of the film for me was the expression on each child's face when the doctors turned on the device for the first time.

The kids were portrayed as happy in the family background stories. They were shown playing in school and with their friends in their neighborhood. They went on family vacations. It certainly appeared to me that all of the children with hearing loss were having very worthwhile and enjoyable lives.

However, the first time the children heard their parents' voices, an immeasurable glow appeared in their eyes. As I watched, I started crying. At the time, I attributed my tears to the new connection they were making with their parents. I thought about what a great gift those families were receiving.

People from the hard of hearing community explained why they would want to self-segregate to make accommodations easier and build kinship. But after seeing the movie, I still didn't understand why anyone within the hearing loss community wouldn't want to have the magic of sound brought to them by any means necessary.

Looking back on it now, I realize that I had never completely internalized there being a real option for me to own a fully functioning organic or artificial pair of legs. My failed experiences with prosthestics and my physical deficits kept me from ever believing that could be an option.

A few years back, I was speaking at a convention where durable medical equipment providers were promoting their latest technology. Stan, a sales rep for one of the large prosthesis manufacturers, approached me after my presentation and told me that he really enjoyed my program. After speaking to his manager, Stan said they were interested in sponsoring me as a representative of their company.

They explained that they had developed an innovative design for a computerized knee and foot combination and were looking for a double amputee to try out their new system. I shared my experience with the old legs I used back in school and the many challenges I had. Both gentlemen assured me that it would be different now. "Things have come a long way. We are going to get you up and running without the assistance of crutches or canes."

They took photos and measurements of my legs. We were looking at different foot designs. They even took me to a shoe store to show me what styles of shoes would work best on the different feet.

I was surprised about how excited I was with the possibility of having legs. I even spoke to members of my family to share my newfound hopes about the potential for me to be able to walk. They all warned me, "Don't get your hopes up."

I tried to remain cautiously optimistic. Then, all of a sudden, I had visions of being tall and what that would mean for me. I began to envision myself carrying something in my arms, and moving at the same time effortlessly. I would be able to walk and hold hands with a significant other no matter the terrain. I saw myself kissing a woman, while I was standing. Then, I was dancing the tango!

But then, I began to wonder something entirely different. I wondered, *If I am able to get these legs and gain the ability to walk, would my friends still be my friends?*

When I played wheelchair basketball, there was one guy on my team that always said, "If I ever regain the use of my legs and can walk again, I'll never talk to any of you losers again."

His hurtful attitude would make his disappearance not that big of a loss for us. But it did make me wonder how people might change if they actually *overcame their disability*.

Once I asked a girlfriend if she would be able to stay with me if I ever gained the ability to walk. She said, "Being able to walk is a pretty big deal. I never really wanted to tell you that because, if you did ever experience it firsthand, it would show you what you have been missing. It could change what makes you the person you are."

She continued, "I don't know who the new Matt would be. I would have to see who and what you become before I could tell you if I would stay."

It turns out, we would never have to learn. Not too long after I started the conversations with Stan, he came back to me with the bad news. "After the engineers reviewed the measurements of your little legs and analyzed the x-rays of your hips, you are not a good candidate for our new prosthesis."

We had only been talking for a few weeks. But I had already started imagining myself walking. As with any major emotional loss, I went through a mourning phase for the potential of something I never thought I would be able to do. I was quite sad for a few days. I tried to forget about it and put those feelings away so I could get back to living.

The reason they gave me for not being a good candidate was that the physical characteristics of my little legs didn't meet the specifications for their products.

Of course, I was born without a traditional leg structure. But more than that, where my leg bone attaches to my pelvis, I do not have a ball and socket joint. The end of the rounded bone attaches directly to the socket without the benefit of the ball.

I have movement and feeling in my legs, but I lack some of the full range of mo-tion and flexibility. The best way I can explain it is this: when I am riding a horse in a western saddle, it is painful for me because my little legs don't bend out sideways as far as those of a traditional person's legs do.

The overall short length of my legs is also a problem. The most effective prosthesis users have longer bones and knees to which they attach the adaptive equipment. A leg is basically a lever; the longer the lever, the more power you can generate and the more control you can have.

At the time of my evaluation for the new prosthesis, I had been sitting for over thirty-five years. That position caused in my back a bit of a natural, rolling curve, which they claimed would prevent me from achieving a full, upright posture while standing.

Offering hope, the engineers told me, "In the near future, doctors will have poten-tial solutions to your challenges. They could reconstruct both of your leg bones and add ball and socket joints to your hips. They could rebuild your back. You would have to participate in several years of physical therapy to learn how to walk with the new technology - after they produce it."

Of course, technology is advancing every day. Someday, there may be something I could use to achieve a traditional walking gait and upright posture. But it would have to be better than what I am doing now with my wheelchair for me to pursue it. It would not only be a big physical change, but also a huge mental one.

POINT TO PONDER: Have you ever had something you never knew you wanted but always did, only to have it taken away?

The knowledge of my own uniqueness leads me to believe that I can accomplish almost anything. To do so within the society in which I exist is indeed the best way for me to be accepted and become successful. My identity is the positive story I tell myself about who I am, developed from all my knowledge and experiences.

For decades, I have been living my life trying to be something that I am not. I falsely believed that I was an able-bodied person with simply with more challenges than most people.

Now, I know differently. I understand that "I am disabled."

CHAPTER 5

A New Understanding

ven after recognizing that I am disabled, the hardest parts of my life are when people treat me like I am disabled. Able-bodied culture and the physical environments in which I exist are the things that define & make me as disabled.

However, my new understanding of how my disability impacts other people encourages me to seek out and work harder to understand how to relieve the uncomfortable moments for everyone and myself. I still have to integrate myself into society as best as I can.

That means I am constantly living and grappling with the disabling contradiction of who I know I am when I am alone versus how I appear and exist in other people's minds. I know I am complete, but I feel as if strangers see me as half a man. Even friends will say things like, "Imagine how great you could have been if you had legs."

Will my feelings of inadequacy ever be soothed? Will society see me as complete? In my basic constitution of who I am, I feel like I have to immediately tell people what I am missing and what I have.

"Hi, my name is Matt Glowacki. I was born without any legs, but everything else is there and it works just fine."

It's both sad and rather funny to me that I have gotten so good at this. I can introduce myself to someone and answer the next two questions that enter their mind simultaneously. "Why doesn't he have legs?" and "I wonder if he has a penis?"

I watch people seamlessly fit into a crowd and I become jealous. There is never a time when I don't at least feel like I have something to prove or that I am not in some way part of the show. I can easily fall into the victim mentality when thinking like this. There's nothing I can do about not having any legs. There's nothing I can do about people underestimating my abilities, feeling sorry for me, or viewing me as only "half" a person.

Almost every day when I'm traveling to speak somewhere, I still have to use a public bathroom without being able to close the stall door for privacy. I find myself constantly having to risk my life by pushing my wheelchair down city streets without curb cuts, looking at how to get back to the safety of a sidewalk. Complete strangers judge me as incompetent and incomplete simply because I don't have legs and use a wheelchair.

When people tell me all the reasons I don't have to do something, it makes me not want to try. The more I disengage because it is hard or I don't feel like trying, the more it keeps me from being able to succeed.

A friend of mine once told me, "Victims can succeed, but people who see themselves as victims never will."

I have found that defining myself as a victim and letting that identity dictate who I am and what I can do is selling myself short. I choose to be noticed for the work I do, the things I enjoy, and what I am able to contribute. By embracing my challenges and finding my own happiness, others are able to see me as attractive, positive, and inspired.

Now as I write this, I am content. I have accepted who I am, who I am not, and who I intend to be. They are all solidly grounded in the same person.

I just wish it wouldn't have taken me forty-four years to get here.

In many of the question-and-answer portions of my presentations, people have asked, "When did you realize you didn't have legs, and how did you deal with that?"

For forty-three of those years, I responded by saying, "I don't know that I ever have become aware of it."

I was living in denial, both for myself and for other people. I did my best to ignore all of my outward differences. I created my own blind spots in how I saw myself.

I finally realized I'm disabled, and I've finally made peace with it (or I'm making peace with it). Just because we the disabled aren't like the majority doesn't mean that we are any less or should be treated any differently.

We know you can see us, because we see you. We have to—every day. Know that the world is as much ours as it is yours.

For every human being you meet, turn, face them, and interact with them, no matter how they're put together. Humanity comes in all kinds of packages.

"When green is all there is to be,
It could make you wonder why, but why wonder?
Why wonder, I am green and it'll do fine, it's beautiful!
And I think it's what I want to be."
Kermit D. Frog

Made in the USA
Monee, IL
28 September 2023

43591054R00105